PUBLIC HEALTH IN THE 21ST CENTURY

EMOTIONALITY OF COVID-19. NOW AND AFTER

THE WAR AGAINST A VIRUS

MAXIMILIANO KORSTANJE
AND
ADRIAN SCRIBANO
EDITORS

nova
Medicine & Health
New York

NOTICE TO THE READER

The Publisher has taken reasonable care in the preparation of this book, but makes no expressed or implied warranty of any kind and assumes no responsibility for any errors or omissions. No liability is assumed for incidental or consequential damages in connection with or arising out of information contained in this book. The Publisher shall not be liable for any special, consequential, or exemplary damages resulting, in whole or in part, from the readers' use of, or reliance upon, this material. Any parts of this book based on government reports are so indicated and copyright is claimed for those parts to the extent applicable to compilations of such works.

Independent verification should be sought for any data, advice or recommendations contained in this book. In addition, no responsibility is assumed by the Publisher for any injury and/or damage to persons or property arising from any methods, products, instructions, ideas or otherwise contained in this publication.

This publication is designed to provide accurate and authoritative information with regard to the subject matter covered herein. It is sold with the clear understanding that the Publisher is not engaged in rendering legal or any other professional services. If legal or any other expert assistance is required, the services of a competent person should be sought. FROM A DECLARATION OF PARTICIPANTS JOINTLY ADOPTED BY A COMMITTEE OF THE AMERICAN BAR ASSOCIATION AND A COMMITTEE OF PUBLISHERS.

Additional color graphics may be available in the e-book version of this book.

Library of Congress Cataloging-in-Publication Data

ISBN: 978-1-53619-534-7

Published by Nova Science Publishers, Inc. † New York

CONTENTS

Foreword: **COVID-19, Anger and the Neoliberal Society 2020** **vii**
Freddy Timmermann

Preface **xiii**

Chapter 1 The Dilemmas of the Lockdown: A Society in Post COVID-19 Days **1**
Maximiliano E. Korstanje

Chapter 2 The Hunger Games: A Look at Food Interventions in the Context of Covid-19 **11**
Adrian Scribano and Aldana Boragnio

Chapter 3 The Enemy Inside **39**
Primavera Fisogni

Chapter 4 Pandemic, Internet and Emotions: Politics of Sensibilities and Commodification of Audiences **59**
Pedro Lisdero and Marion Fonrouge

Chapter 5 Economic, Social and Psychological Issues of Survival in the Pandemic: The Case of Russian Federation **83**
Irina Burak and Tatiana Razumova

Chapter 6	Long Live to the Urban Flesh *Fabio La Rocca*	**107**
Chapter 7	Pandemic, Social Policies and Emotions in the Metropolitan Area of Buenos Aires *Angélica De Sena*	**125**
Chapter 8	Sensibilities of Eating Inside: Emotions and Food Practices in a Time of a Pandemic *Aldana Boragnio*	**151**
Chapter 9	Die Alone in Argentina: A View from Sensibilities in Times of the Pandemic *Adrián Scribano and Jorge Duperré*	**173**
About the Authors		**197**
About the Editors		**203**
Index		**205**

Foreword

COVID-19, ANGER AND THE NEOLIBERAL SOCIETY 2020

Freddy Timmermann
University Bernardo de O´Higgins, Santiago de Chile, Chile

The recent virus outbreak recently originated in Wuhan, China not only grids the global trade into a halt but also evinces the material asymmetries and inequalities of neoliberal economic policies worldwide (Zizek, 2019; Mair, 2020; Wallace et al. 2020). In Latin America and particularly in Chile, this global pandemic shows its destructive power potentiated by decades of (neo)liberalism initiated since 1975 and politically perpetuated by a bloody Regime which violated all fundamental rights. This period of violence and fear certainly cemented a rampant individualism which maximizes pleasure through the consuming-machine (Timmermann 2019). In the political sphere, neoliberalism paved the ways for certain political stability which was not based on the consensus but on the lack of interests in politics. The social life, so to speak, succumbed to the macro-economic liberal reasoning.

The end of 90s decade witnesses a clear –if not irreversible-disillusionment for the partisan political parties and professional politicians who are seen as a ruling elite disinterested for the citizens´ demands. As a result of this, the stability dotted by the Chilean political parties sets the pace to the rise of new discontents that places the political order in jeopardy. The neoliberal society characterizes by high levels of fragmentation and social decomposition which leads gradually to an excess of consumption (widely shaped in social maladies as drug-addiction, obesity, alcoholism, and crime). To put the same in other terms, President Sebastian Piñera was scarcely elected president with only 27% of Chilean voters. The anger seems to occupy a central position in this foreword I love to write for my good friends and colleagues Adrian Scribano & Maximiliano E. Korstanje.

The foreword brings some reflection to the philosophical quandary of anger which results from a previous offence when one of the affected victims has no possibility of retaliation. As Martha Nussbaum puts it, there is a difference between anger and grief which merits to be discussed. While the former signals to do something (often harm) against the perpetrator, the latter asks for something in return when the victim fells vulnerated. The victim sees she was lost something and seeks restoration to placate the pain. In the case of anger, the damage should be directed against the perpetrator. The problem of anger often associates with the dilemma of justice. The anger potentiates when the perpetrator avoids the punishment or the act of retaliation. Under the auspices of some political mechanism, the anger can be temporarily mitigated but it blasts or takes other channels when the victims´ demands are not met. This is exactly what western popular parlance sees in the riots and disturbing events that involved Chile since October of 2019. This discontent includes meagre pensions (which sometimes equates to USD 200), rumours of political corruption, adjoined to pharmaceutical monopolies that offer a market accessible for few people who keep a high purchasing power without mentioning heavy taxes and rates in electricity, and basic services almost impossible to pay. To the political corruption, I can add, several denounces of sexual abuse to children and the protection of the Catholic diocese to the accused priests. Over recent years, the protests combine a legitimate component of the discontented citizen who organizes themselves to present their demands and some illegal gang-bands which take the opportunity to head riots and lootings. For some voices, this coalescence is a clear sign of social decomposition.

The climate of conflictivity which is peacefully re-channeled towards peaceful protest converges with the rise of marginal groups. The policemen violently repress all involving groups. Not only violating the basic rights but also undermining the check and balance institutions proper of the democratic order. There is a type of new communal property destruction which includes bus stations, universities, churches, commercial shopping malls and cars. To put the same in bluntly, the private property which was the quintessential feature of the neoliberal order is now under constant attack. We live a new process of late retaliation (violence) that in some cases transcends the authority of the nation-state. Of course I must confess, all governments and administration make errors in the struggle against the COVID-19. Some governments fall in the error because of technical ignorance or because of indifference to the net of experts, but others overlook systematically the maladies (inequalities) produced by the economic order which finally are exacerbated by the pandemic. I mean preferably to poverty and the crisis of trust of Chilean citizen to the public information which was historically tergiversated in the past to protect the partisan interests. What is more important, the funds assigned to Health ministry for the COVID was 12.000 Chilean pesos. While the pandemic accelerated the long-dormant economic recession, citizens lose their jobs and private firms tittered on the brink of collapse. In the mid of this disaster and serious economic downturn, local mayors unilaterally increase their salaries (almost 40 or 50%) while parliament diets are reduced to 25%. This lack of coherence and coordinated efforts leads citizenship to face an unparalleled state of anxiety and fear as never before. What is worse, the sanitary information and cooperation obscure more than they clarify. Communication process not only seems to be poor but based on ongoing contradictions. In this respect, Piñera boasts that Chile has successfully remained the infections relatively stable, controlling the curve of new cases, while the Education ministry devotes efforts in getting the students back to schools. However, on the streets, there is the reign of the confusion and the ambiguous liberality of the managerial perspective.

Several streets in urban cities as Santiago are overcrowded while mass-consumption and the celebrations are being held Chile-wide. Every family had a member who violates the lockdown to work. Not surprisingly the economic deterioration is accompanied by populist neoliberal policies oriented to protect the economist interests of the ruling elite. Once again, the COVID-19 shows not only the financial asymmetries generated by neoliberal agenda but the suspension of the *social contract* of society. In a post COVID-19 context, I see with extreme clarity the vulnerability of community in view of the corporative interests of a political elite which lacks legitimacy. The government amounts the spectacle of Disaster only to preserve the status quo while running the risk of releasing the Kraken; last but not least, the global pandemic not only reveals the miseries of the neoliberal discourse, as well as the political contradiction of the national liberalism. As Korstanje (2018) puts it, neoliberalism rests on shaky foundations and contradictions when it equates to national liberalism simply because the sense of nationhood and the nation-states contradict the essence of liberal choice –or so to say the autonomy of the man-. I finally want to celebrate critical approaches -like Scribano & Korstanje´s book-that helps to strip out neoliberalism from its sacred veil of the sainthood. Last but not least, I wish to thank Professor Maximiliano Korstanje for the edition and proofread of the present short foreword.

References

Korstanje, M. E. (2018). *The Challenges of democracy in the War on terror: the liberal state before the advance of terrorism.* Abingdon, Routledge.

Mair, S. (2020). Neoliberal economics, planetary health, and the COVID-19 pandemic: a Marxist ecofeminist analysis. *The Lancet Planetary Health*, *4*(12), e588-e596.

Nussbaum M (2016) *Anger and forgiveness: resentment, generosity and justice.* Oxford, Oxford University Press.

Timmermann F. (2019) "Fear and Wrath: the neoliberal civilization of Chile from 1990 to 2019. In *Allegories of a never-ending war.* Korstanje Mm. (ed), Hauppauge, Nova Science Pubs.

Zizek, S. (2020). *PANDEMIC!: Covid-19 Shakes the World.* New York, John Wiley & Sons.

PREFACE

Similarly to the attacks on the World Trade Center on September 11 of 2001, a foundational event that marked the turn of the century, the recent virus outbreak in Wuhan, China resonates heavily in the social imaginary of West. Both events have differences and of course commonalities. 9/11 epitomizes the struggle of Western civilization against an invisible enemy, terrorism, while now the target is a virus. Both emulate the doctrine of living with the enemy inside. Another commonality rests on the fact the same transport means that facilitate the state of emergency are paradoxically and at the same time mainly victims. Based on the invitation of well-renowned experts coming from four continents, the present book discusses critically the effects of COVID-19 as well as the global pandemic in society. To some extent, experts and colleagues of all pundits energetically emphasize the economic crisis of COVID-19 overlooking the durable effects in the societal background. This book intends to fill the gap giving a fresh insight which explains the role of social distancing and the lockdown in a new emerging society. Although chapters can be read separately, they are finely grounded into a common argumentation, as the pandemic affirms not only the geopolitical tensions of what Scambler dubbed as a fractured society but also starts a feudalization process where the Spectacle of Death prevails.

Chapter 1 - This preliminary chapter introduces readers to the content of the book; so to speak an editorial project oriented to discuss the durable effects of the global pandemic (COVID-19) in society. Although a whole portion of studies, books and publications aimed at exploring the economic consequences of the virus, less attention was given to the social maladies – i.e., racist and separatist discourses, violence and phobias- the COVID-19 certainly generates. The COVID-19 potentiates the fear of stranger closing the West in a philosophical dilemma. All restrictions and travel bans that nation-states dispose for stopping the contagion inscribe into a process that political scientists know as the "securitization process". The present chapter holds the thesis that COVID-19 affirms a tendency originated in 9/11 which accelerates the death of hospitality. In the new normality, the "Other" has become an *undesired guest.*

Chapter 2 - Since government actions at all levels began in relation to the COVID-19 pandemic in Argentina, the State, the market and NGOs have been targeted at the poorest and most impoverished sectors of the country. Based on the analysis and interpretation of various records of the mass media and official documents, this article systematizes various difficulties around hunger, with the aim of opening a critical discussion on them from the perspective of sociologies of bodies/emotions. The expository strategy will be as follows: a) the theoretical starting point of the connection between hunger, the body and emotions is synthesized, b) the situation of poverty and pre-pandemic hunger in Argentina is outlined, c) some of the multiple emotions of the intervention are characterized and d) some interpretations of the interventions characterized are presented.

Chapter 3 - The global world has recently been under attack from a new enemy, whose microscopic shape shuttered every aspect of human life: health, relations, social and economic frames. The COVID-19 outbreak can be compared to a war, with relation to the number of victims made worldwide. Still unknown in its several biological aspects, Coronavirus is currently going to update the concept of enemy. As the author intends to argue, the pandemic brought to the forefront the idea of *enemy as an insider which* constantly *interacts with the host*. The enemy can be attacked only assuming it, making it part of both the individual body and the social body. According to this perspective immunization cannot be seen in terms of an exemption but properly as an inclusion. The author's reasoning starts from a short account of the classic paradigm of friend/enemy sketched by Schmitt (1932) and developed by Vitale (1992) in order to show the novelty of the 'enemy inside.' Then the author will take in consideration the processes that give rise to immunization, through the lens of General System Thinking (Urbani Ulivi, 2019) that better fit the purpose to explore such a complex topic. The author reaches the conclusion that immunization makes the enemy (virus) and the host (the biological substratum) adversaries: this dynamic, by reducing the dangerous potential of enemy, puts it under control. Thus, any process of immunization can be interpreted as the making of a community, differently from Esposito's theory (1998; 2001) of a sharp distinction between *immunitas* and *communitas* (immunity/community).

Chapter 4 - On March 11, 2019, the World Health Organization declared the status of a pandemic for the rapid expansion of COVID-19. In a short period of time, the daily lives of billions of people around the world would never be the same: the successive strategies that were adopted in different countries implied significant changes in most of the subjects' daily experiences, from the way of working to the family relationship itself. Most of the situations of interactions in the context of the pandemic are carried out in virtual contexts, and specifically through social networks. Thus, COVID-19 is imposed as a recurring "topic of discussion": WhatsApp groups, Facebook, etc. are filled with messages and discussions about it. Thinking in terms of social research, it is possible to imagine a Big Data strategy to analyze the traceability of messages, and to map the density of the circulation of information. However, it is also possible to ask ourselves some questions that seek the qualitative meanings of the practice of receiving and re-sending messages related to the subject, while taking into account its relationship with their form. In this direction, the objective of this chapter is to analyze the emotions linked to the interactions in social networks associated with COVID-19. To do this, the authors applied a self-administered survey to 307 respondents in 17 European countries, selected using the snowball sampling technique between March 17th and April

18th, where the authors inquired about how people feel when they receive/send information related to the pandemic. Given the multiple possible interpretations, the authors are interested in linking some discussions around digital labor, that is, the ability of social networks to market to an audience. This means emphasizing one of the ways these media have, in the framework of the renewed and massive situations of digital interaction, of capturing people's energies and transforming them into merchandise (Fuchs, 2014). The analysis focuses on the fact that what is commercialized is the willingness to be part of a group that receives messages, so it is not enough to just know the quantifiable dimension of the action of forwarding, but also what is at stake is the relationship between the objective field and the willingness of the subjects to be part of these audiences. Therefore, beyond the re-production of the practice (whether it is re-sent or not re-sent), the authors are interested here in exploring how the qualitative sense that agents give to it could be associated with policies of digital sensibilities (Scribano and Lisdero, 2019). That is, perceptions framed in specific regimes of sensibilities that allow connecting bodily geometries with grammars of action (Scribano, 2017) that have a specific support and content in the digital field. This allows us to advance in the description of "platform sensibilities" as a sign of the ongoing social structuration processes.

Chapter 5 - This chapter contains the broad economic and social review of the COVID-19 consequences which Russian Federation faces today. COVID-19 epidemic update had a great impact on all spheres, people's lives had changed dramatically: many people have contracted the illness, others lost their jobs and incomes, almost all were overcome with panic. So, the main objective of the Russian Government was to rapidly develop a program of urgent response in the sphere of healthcare as well as in preventing deep negative consequences in decrease of peoples' incomes and welfare. The special measures of economic and social support were undertaken by the government towards SMEs and people under great risks of poverty. Volunteers' activities aimed at care of elderly people under the isolation restrictions became widely developed. To prevent the risk of contamination lots of people in different spheres were urged to work distantly, this process was supported by wide access to informational technologies and equipment and well-developed skills of specialists. Still, for many companies it was a severe challenge which required training of personnel and new management tools. During the isolation period distant professional learning was of great importance and popularity: it helped to prepare people to overcome the crisis with marketable knowledge and skills.

Chapter 6 - In the present chapter the authors bring some reflection about changes of the current reconfigured urban space and the orientation of a revaluated vision of ecosophy with some specific elements of the ambiance that the authors can observe in the daily experience. With this structure, the authors build in their way a kind of sensible thought to elucidate a vision of some forms of urban social dimension. The authors' intention in this hot-debate aims to show some fragments constructing a particular vision of the spirit of the time in order to analyze the actual socio-urban dimension. In this perspective, will bring together some goals as the illustration of the actual city, the experience in the post COVID-19 situation, the idea of proximity, the new vision of ecological sensibility, where each of them encloses other peculiars aspects of the authors' experience of the social urban world.

Chapter 7 - The Metropolitan Area of Buenos Aires is one of the poorest areas of Argentina. In this area is located La Matanza, the largest geographic municipality with the largest population and greatest vulnerability, as indicated by data from a pre-pandemic investigation. In March 2020, in Argentina the "social, preventive and mandatory isolation" was declared in the face of the Covid-19 pandemic, which meant an increase in poverty and social assistance. In this context, an online survey study was carried out (in four waves: April, May, June and September/October) in order to ascertain the changes in the poverty situation of the population of La Matanza among the people receiving a social benefit, and related emotions around the pandemic and their own situation of vulnerability. For this, the exposition of the article will be: a) a review of the social and economic situation of the territory in question pre-pandemic; b) development of the theoretical perspective regarding social policies to address poverty in connection with emotions, considering social interventions that construct meanings, elaborate perceptions, and are located in the performativity of the aforementioned policies; c) development of the methodological aspects of research and analysis of quantitative information, taking into account the population that receives a social program and the emotions that emerge in relation to the pandemic. In this way, this chapter aims to make a substantial contribution to understanding the impact on the sensitivities of the recipients of the social interventions implemented in the context of a pandemic.

Chapter 8 - In the pandemic situation, where social distancing and confinement were presented as the main tools for its prevention, eating became confined to the inside of the home. For those who have a home to stay in, eating has been reinstated as a practice in the private sphere and as a need to be met while remaining indoors. Eating is a daily practice that produces and reproduces the body, and it is shaped from habits, norms and customs that are expressed in social sensibilities. At the same time, it is directly linked to the configuration of emotions as the body/food/ hunger/emotions relationship unfolds in an unbreakable continuum. While the diet is configured as a set of practices that are practices of the politics of sensibilities, food and commensality practices imply and express sociabilities and experiences. In this case, by knowing about diet, food practices and commensality, the authors will know how people put into practice specific knowledge about food to organize and regulate the planning, preparation and consumption of their daily meals in the context of isolation and of a new organization of time. Thus, knowing about diet and its practices will allow us to know the sensibilities and experiences in the context of a pandemic, where food practices take on a greater importance, since it highlights not only the possibilities of access, variation, diversification and consumption, but specific sensibilities around cooking, eating and the home. The objective of this chapter is to expose the sensibilities of eating in a time of pandemic in Argentina and Spain, based on a comparative study between the two countries. To do this, the authors conducted an online survey, self-administered during the first five weeks of isolation and confinement, and in-depth interviews with young people from the tenth week, seeking to discover the eating practices of isolation in articulation with the time/space relationship, which are configured from a politics of sensibilities as cognitive-affective practices of feeling in the pandemic world.

Chapter 9 - The objective of this work is to reflect on the sensibilities related to dying and death, in the context of the current coronavirus pandemic. The presentational strategy that the authors have envisaged in this regard begins by defining and establishing the theoretical perspective in which the authors' proposal is framed: the sociology of bodies/emotions. Then the authors go back to another global crisis that occurred a century ago, known as the Spanish Flu. The reason for this is to recover some antecedents that allow us to enrich the authors' approach to this phenomenon that is still ongoing; not in comparable terms (since both episodes are not), but rather illustrative. Finally, the authors will deal with the three traits that, in their opinion, characterize the collective bond with the dying and corpses at the present moment: mediated death, regulated death, and cherished death.

In: Emotionality of COVID-19 ISBN: 978-1-53619-534-7
Editors: M. Korstanje and S. Adrian © 2021 Nova Science Publishers, Inc.

Chapter 1

The Dilemmas of the Lockdown: A Society in Post COVID-19 Days

***Maximiliano E. Korstanje*[1,2,*]**
[1]University of Palermo, Argentina
[2]CERS, University of Leeds, Leeds LS2 9JT, UK

Abstract

This preliminary chapter introduces readers to the content of the book; so to speak an editorial project oriented to discuss the durable effects of the global pandemic (COVID-19) in society. Although a whole portion of studies, books and publications aimed at exploring the economic consequences of the virus, less attention was given to the social maladies – i.e., racist and separatist discourses, violence and phobias- the COVID-19 certainly generates. The COVID-19 potentiates the fear of stranger closing the West in a philosophical dilemma. All restrictions and travel bans that nation-states dispose for stopping the contagion inscribe into a process that political scientists know as the "securitization process". The present chapter holds the thesis that COVID-19 affirms a tendency originated in 9/11 which accelerates the death of hospitality. In the new normality, the "Other" has become an *undesired guest.*

---

* Corresponding Author's E-mail: mkorst@palermo.edu.

Keywords: Death of Hospitality, West, COVID-19, Terror, Society

1. INTRODUCTION

The COVID-19 left incalculable financial losses, as well as human deceases, changing not only the geopolitics but gridding the global trade into an unparalleled halt (Sheridan et al. 2020). The global pandemic shocks directly the world while evincing the material asymmetries and inequalities culturally enrooted in the postmodern capitalism (Ali, Asaria and Stranges 2020; Matthewman and Huppatz, 2020; Black 2020). Sociology of COVID-19 remains in its infancy. Some voices alert on the end of capitalism, at least as we know it (Zizek 2020). To date, it is very hard to precise the evolution of the pandemic. At the end of December of 2019, the Western audience captivated by the news coming from China revolving around a new virus outbreak originated in Wuhan city. Doubtless, this new virus, which is known as SARSCOv2, gradually becomes in a global pandemic infecting more than 93 million peoples and causing more than two millions of deaths (numbers updated at 15 January of 2021).

Although governments suddenly disposed of radical measures such as the closure of borders, airspace without mentioning the imposition of strict lockdowns the virus showed higher transmissibility. Over the recent decades, the West faced similar crises associated with SARS, Ebola and Swine Flu, but nothing like COVID-19 (Richardson et al. 2017). The virus disseminates rapidly because of the mobile infrastructure of the Western Hemisphere which connects far-away cities in hours, as well as the overcrowding that characterizes the urban areas (Adey et al. 2014; Lapointe 2020). To enumerate some mediate consequences of the pandemic we come across with discourses of racism or chauvinism directed against Asian tourists (Mostafanezhad and Cheer 2020), geopolitical tensions (Lee and Haupt 2020), without mentioning political crisis and turmoil derived from the economic crisis (Rogerson and Baum 2020).

The mass transport means, as well as the tourist travels, were the key factors that allowed a rapid propagation of the virus worldwide. Although sociologists and colleagues of different pundits have captivated by the advance of COVID-19, less was known about its aftermaths. Sociologists are often educated to study social phenomena in normal conditions, but few voices are experts in *disaster studies.* As Enrico Quarantelli puts it, a disaster denotes the idea that the normal conditions of existence that make the life possible in society are temporal suspended or simply disappeared. Any state of disaster speaks of the incapacity of society to give a valid response to external or internal danger, in which case the social order is in jeopardy. The question of whether of disaster interrogates furtherly our vulnerability as well as the existent deficiencies to deal with urgent matters. In fact, post-disaster manuals never apply at the best as they were written when the disaster takes hit (Quarantelli 1988; 1997; 1998). Of course, this is the case of COVID-19. The invitation of a leading worldly publisher as Nova Science Publisher to edit a book with a focus on COVID-19 was a brilliant idea we – jointly to Argentinean philosopher Adrian Scribano- will not waste. Also, we started to work in the selection of authors who come from different latitudes and cultures. To avoid the Anglo-centrism which marks the pace in social science, we invited scholars who are not native English speaker. This seems to have some limitations because of the grammar barriers, but we bet it worth our times. The present (short) chapter discusses the long-durable effects of COVID-19 in society while discussing the different chapters that form the present book while lays the foundations towards new paradigms to understand the effects of the pandemic in postmodern society.

2. COVID-19, SOCIETY AND POLITICS

In a seminal paper, which entitles *sociology of COVID-19,* Steve Matthewman and Kate Huppatz (2020) locates the COVID-19 in the epicenter of the most serious health and economic crisis of human history. Global citizens who were accustomed to travel across the globe were suddenly immersed in a new social experiment where their basic rights to circulate freely were radically altered by the governments. The pandemic is changing human relationships, reciprocities and emotions and of course the ways of making sociology; so to speak, different social maladies already existent in the late capitalism – far from being resolved- become more acute in the post COVID-19 context. Sociologists should re-imagine the infrastructure of a new social world based on social distancing, lockdowns and indifference by the "Other". In this vein, Korstanje and George (2020) called the attention to the shifts in the travel behavior as well as in the ways the alterity is imagined in Western civilization. The scientific expedition that inspired the rise of sociology and anthropology started from the needs of "being there" to study the natives. The "Other", for better or worse, was an object of curiosity which should be subordinated to the scientific gaze. In the days after 9/11, the "Other" is seen as an undesired guest, a potential enemy who looms to attack anytime and anywhere. In the post 9/11 days, anyone could be a potential terrorist while just after COVID-19 all us are potential (terrorists) carriers of a lethal disease. Without any doubt, the world is experiencing a feudalization process where the national borders are in constant tension and negotiation but far from being a foundational event, COVID-19 closes a process initiated after 9/11. In that process, the *Non-Western "Other"* is suspected to be a future enemy, neglected and exiled through the scrutiny of modern surveillance. In a nutshell, authors hold the polemic thesis that Western hospitality is dying by the introduction of a fear culture to govern the workforce (Korstanje and George 2020). In consonance with this, Geoffrey Pleyers (2020) acknowledges that the pandemic affirms the authority emanating from the classic nation-states in detriment of the global forces. Having said this, political scientists deal with the risks the world witnesses the emergence of populist leaders who foster nationalist discourse. As he eloquently notes, while the nations closed their borders, citizens looked inside their countries in quest of security and protection. As a result of this, international institutions titter in the brink of collapse. The consequences of COVID-19 entail various geopolitical disputes accompanied by authoritarian guidelines for protection. Everything is allowed in the state of exception. Last but not least, social psychologists Lee Monaghan (2020) continues the discussion left by Scambler who coins the term *fractured society* to explain the inter-class (group) social conflict or tensions -in this case- generated because of COVID-19. Departing from Klein´s concept *disaster capitalism,* Monaghan argues convincingly that COVID-19 finally corroded the basis of human solidarity that was previously affected by the neoliberal agenda, in so doing, some social maladies that characterized liberal society abruptly surfaced.

This book, as stated, combines different theories, and conceptual frameworks giving fresh insights into the effects of COVID-19 in modern society. If this represents the end or a re-start of capitalism only God knows, but what is insure is that the pandemic fractures human relations as never before paving the ways for the emergence of a new society based on the Spectacle of death. The "Other´s death" becomes mainly a factor of cultural entertainment for the global audience worldwide (Tumarkin 2005; Howie 2012; Korstanje 2016; 2018).

3. How to Read This Book

Chapters organized in the present editorial collection can be read separately but they are integrated into a common-thread argument: the consequences of the pandemic in the different micro-sociological spheres of daily life. As remarked, the invited authors who are experts in their fields have no English as their native tongue. The main goal of this book aims to describe how COVID-19 confronts with the Anglo-Saxon cosmology of the world. In so doing, the lens of authors plays a leading role to reconstruct the foundations to new critical sociology in ever-changing capitalism.

As the previous backdrop, the foreword elegantly, which is written by Freddy Timmermann-Lopez, interrogates furtherly the role played by *anger* in the constitution of the neoliberal agenda. Per his viewpoint, neoliberalism started with Allende´s coup and the access of Augusto Pinochet to the presidency of Chile in 1975. Politically speaking, the climate of fear imposed by Pinochet not only paved the ways for the political disinterest but also facilitated the worker union dismantling. The recent protest and social discontent that destabilizes Piñera´s administration comes from a belated retaliation resulted from decades of oppression. The private property which was the quintessential feature of the neoliberal order is now under attack. The recent virus outbreak (COVID-19) activates old-fashioned (authoritarian) practices and dispositions such as the curfew or, army-force patrolling originally characteristic of Pinochet´s Regime.

In the second chapter, Adrian Scribano discusses the interplay of hunger and the sociology of bodies (emotions) in the context of COVID-19. He focuses his analysis on the pre-pandemic situation in Argentina which associates to a much deeper market stagnation, unemployment and perpetual economic crisis. Scribano holds the thesis that – far from being part of the solution, NGOs, the state and the market are allies who have disposed of the citizens´ bodies to manage a climate of scarcity and exploitation. The struggle for containing the virus propagation alludes to a *bellicose metaphor,* the war against a virus!

Primavera Fisogni, in the third chapter, brings some reflections on the doctrine of living with the enemy in, which was originally forged by counter-terrorism experts. His chapter dissects the problem of West to understand the "Alterity", as a potential enemy – like the virus- living within. Her reasoning comes from the model friend-enemy in Carl Schmitt who has molded modern politics. As she puts it, the immunization makes the enemy (the virus) and the host adversaries. In this respect, any process of immunization disciplines the virus keeping it under the human control.

In this vein, Pedro Lisdero and Marion Fonrouge alert on the durable effects of the pandemic in society. To the problem of the internal enemy debated in an earlier chapter, this fourth one adds a more than innovating insight, the big data models and the digital platforms oriented to scrutinize daily social interaction.

These researchers find that the same technology used to follow up the traceability of messages, discussions revolving around COVID-19 paradoxically commoditizes its users.

In the fifth chapter, Irina Burak and Tatiana Razumova expose the study case of the Russian Federation. From different angles, they review the negative effects of COVID-19 in the Russian Federation. The COVID-19 teaches us three sad realities, some people simply die (when their conditions aggravate), some lose their jobs and others may panic. The government adopted not only restrictive measures but also launched to bail out citizens and private companies. The digital technology allowed social distancing as well as the home office in the entire federation. Resiliency will occupy a central position in the economic recovery of the Russian Federation.

In the sixth chapter, Fabio la Rocca explores the archetype of the urban landscapes (the city) in the context of social distancing. As he eloquently notes, the face of the city has been radically transformed by the restrictive measures adopted by Western states. The city, which historically was a site of connection, now becomes in a space of eradication. He coins the term *the desert city* to symbolize the days of lockdown in different in Europe. It is safe to say that the extension of the interior in our apartments was exteriorized beyond the window to recreate a social manifestation of tribal reciprocity during the COVID-19. While forcefully constrained to stay safer at home, lay-citizens get out balconies to interact with "the Other".

Angelica de Sena, in the seventh chapter, shows the grim future of La Matanza, one of the poorest and largest regions of Buenos Aires Metropolitan area. When President Alberto Fernandez decided to impose the lockdown it generated devastating effects for citizens who witnessed how the economy plummeted. She conducts some online surveys to describe the emotions of La Matanza´s dwellers. The obtained outcomes reveal that fear, and anxiety followed by boredom and worry are the main axes of what consulted people normally feel as long as the COVID-19.

In the eighth chapter, Aldana Boragnio proffers a more than interesting diagnosis about COVID-19 and the needs to be safe at home. For those who are forced to stay at home, the act of eating becomes a practice of the private domain. As she remarks, eating seems to be a social practice that reproduces the body while framing habits and customs as well as countless social sensibilities. The global pandemic not only alters diets but food practices in different ways. The chapter aims at describing the sensibilities of eating in the post-pandemic days while laying the foundations towards a new understanding of commensality, and the rite of the banquet.

The last chapter -on the ink of Adrian Scribano and Jorge Duperre- draws a comparison between COVID-19 and the Spanish Flu, a virus that whipped humanity in the former century. Authors use the term *present, mediated and cherished death* to explain the disposition of audiences to the spectacle of death, packaged and sold by the mass media. The pandemic suspended and radically changed all funerary rites, stripping out the veil of death from its sainthood. The act of dying accompanied or alone -exiled like Oedipus-, which is the core of the tragedy, seems to be one of the controversial themes this chapter deals with.

CONCLUSION

One of the problems of COVID-19 remains with the fact that we know nothing respecting how this game ends. The chapters lumped together in this volume study the durable effects of COVID-19 in different fields of private or public life. Basically, far from being a turning point, this pandemic seems to affirm the material inequalities and social maladies proper of capitalism which ranges from digital exploitation, to labor precaritization or the introduction of a fear culture as a form of cultural entertainment. What is equally important, our travel behavior and customs changed in the same way how the foreign tourists are treated. Asian tourists not only are feared but discriminated as potential carriers of COVID-19. The national or inter-estate borders have been re-drawn in view of a new politics where the “Other” is the enemy – if not the terrorist- (Korstanje 2017). Whatever the case may be, the social distancing as well as the lockdown, recreates the conditions to the rise of new geopolitical disputes, chauvinist discourses, or long-dormant sentiment of separatism. Probably the global economy sets the pace to a more feudalized world where “the Other” becomes in an *undesired guest.* This process does not begin with the pandemic, but with 9/11 and the War on Terror. The virus, so to speak, closes the doors of an epoch I has dubbed as the *End of hospitality*, at least as we know it.

REFERENCES

Adey, P., Bissell, D., Hannam, K., Merriman, P. and Sheller, M. (Eds.). (2014). *The Routledge Handbook of Mobilities*. Abingdon: Routledge.

Ali, S., Asaria, M. and Stranges, S. (2020). COVID-19 and inequality: are we all in this together? *Canadian Journal of Public Health*, 111(3), 415 - 416.

Black, J. (2020). COVID-19 and the Real Impossible. *International Journal of Žižek Studies*, 14(2): 1 - 12.

Howie, L. (2012). *Witnesses to Terror: Understanding the Meanings and Consequences of Terrorism*. New York, Springer.

Klein, N. (2007). *The Shock Doctrine: The Rise of Disaster Capitalism*. London; Macmillan.

Korstanje, M. E. (2016). *The Rise of Thana-Capitalism and Tourism*. Abingdon, Routledge.

Korstanje, M. E. (2017). *Terrorism, Tourism and the End of Hospitality in the West*. New York, Palgrave Macmillan.

Korstanje, M. E. (2018). Dialogues with Slavoj Zizek: Placing the role of torture in context. *International Journal of Žižek Studies*, 12(2): 1 - 7.

Korstanje, M. E. and George, B. (2020). *The Nature and Future of Tourism: a Post COVID-19 Context*. Palm Beach: Apple Academic Press.

Lapointe, D. (2020). Reconnecting tourism after COVID-19: The paradox of alterity in tourism areas. *Tourism Geographies*, 1 - 6.

Lee, J. J. and Haupt, J. P. (2020). Scientific collaboration on COVID-19 amidst geopolitical tensions between the US and China. *The Journal of Higher Education*, 1 - 27.

Matthewman, S. and Huppatz, K. (2020). A sociology of Covid-19. *Journal of Sociology*, 56(4), 675 - 683.

Mostafanezhad, M., Cheer, J. M. and Sin, H. L. (2020). Geopolitical anxieties of tourism:(Im) mobilities of the COVID-19 pandemic. *Dialogues in Human Geography*, 10(2), 182 - 186.

Pleyers, G. (2020). *A Plea for Global Sociology in Times of the Coronavirus.* ISA digital Platform. April 2020. A Global Sociology and the Coronavirus. Available at https://dial.uclouvain.be/pr/boreal/object/ boreal%3A236528/datastream/PDF_01/view.

Quarantelli, E. L. (1988). Disaster crisis management: A summary of research findings. *Journal of management studies*, 25(4), 373 - 385.

Quarantelli, E. L. (1997). Ten criteria for evaluating the management of community disasters. *Disasters*, 21(1), 39 - 56.

Quarantelli, E. L. (Ed.). (1998). *What is a disaster?: Perspectives on the Question*. Psychology Press.

Richardson, E. T., Barrie, M. B., Nutt, C. T., Kelly, J. D., Frankfurter, R., Fallah, M. P. and Farmer, P. E. (2017). The Ebola suspect's dilemma. *The Lancet Global Health*, 5(3), e254 - e256.

Rogerson, C. M. and Baum, T. (2020). COVID-19 and African tourism research agendas. *Development Southern Africa*, 37(5), 727 - 741.

Scambler, G. (2018). *Sociology, Health and the Fractured Society: A Critical Realist Account*. Abingdon: Routledge.

Sheridan, A., Andersen, A. L., Hansen, E. T. and Johannesen, N. (2020). Social distancing laws cause only small losses of economic activity during the COVID-19 pandemic in Scandinavia. *Proceedings of the National Academy of Sciences*, 117(34), 20468 - 20473.

Tumarkin, M. M. (2005). *Traumascapes: The Power and Fate of Places Transformed by Tragedy*. Melbourne, Melbourne Univ. Publishing.

Žižek, S. (2020). *Pandemic! Covid-19 Shakes the World.* New York: OR Books.

In: Emotionality of COVID-19 ISBN: 978-1-53619-534-7
Editors: M. Korstanje and S. Adrian © 2021 Nova Science Publishers, Inc.

Chapter 2

The Hunger Games: A Look at Food Interventions in the Context of Covid-19

Adrian Scribano[1,*], PhD and Aldana Boragnio[2,†], PhD
[1]National Scientific and Technical Research Council (CONICET), Argentina
[2]Center for Research on Consumption, Sensitivities and Creativity (CICSEC), University of Palermo, Argentina

Abstract

Since government actions at all levels began in relation to the COVID-19 pandemic in Argentina, the State, the market and NGOs have been targeted at the poorest and most impoverished sectors of the country. Based on the analysis and interpretation of various records of the mass media and official documents, this article systematizes various difficulties around hunger, with the aim of opening a critical discussion on them from the perspective of sociologies of bodies/emotions. The

* Corresponding Author's E-mail: adrianscribano@gmail.com.
† Corresponding Author's E-mail: boragnio@gmail.com.

expository strategy will be as follows: a) the theoretical starting point of the connection between hunger, the body and emotions is synthesized, b) the situation of poverty and pre-pandemic hunger in Argentina is outlined, c) some of the multiple emotions of the intervention are characterized and d) some interpretations of the interventions characterized are presented.

Keywords: hunger, social interventions, body, emotions

INTRODUCTION

Natural cataclysms, environmental catastrophes, wars, epidemics and pandemics have a common social phenomenon: hunger. Every society, by establishing food production procedures, satiety criteria and the practices of feeling associated with them, somehow establishes a politics of hunger. The political economy associated with capitalism, at least in the last 400 years, set out to be a scientific regulation of scarcity as a "natural phenomenon", generating a system of resource allocation based on unilateral accumulation and a social dispute of systemic adaptation. The state, the market and NGOs are part of the aforementioned processes of managing the scarcity associated with food and hunger. The declaration of social emergency and compulsory isolation immediately impacted the productive structure, labour management and consumption, causing the informality, precariousness and organizational disorganization existing in the country to emerge. Thus, since government actions at all levels began about the COVID-19 pandemic in Argentina, the State, the market and NGOs have made interventions aimed at the poorest and most impoverished sectors of the country. In this context, the present article tries to systematize various interventions around hunger, so as to open a critical discussion about them from the perspective of the sociology of bodies/emotions.

The research strategy and the material that serves as the basis for the analysis and interpretation come from three types of sources: a) records of the mass media and social networks, b) official documents and c) secondary data of other investigations that are being carried out in the Research Centre to which the authors of the article belong. The expository strategy that we have chosen is the following: a) the theoretical starting point of the connection between hunger, the body and emotions are synthesized, b) the situation of poverty and pre-pandemic hunger in the country is outlined, c) some of the emotions that characterize the multiple practices of intervention are outlined, and d) some interpretations are offered about the interventions characterized. The article tries to elaborate a critique of some practices, beyond their legitimacy, of being the product of existing needs, of enjoying political consensus, and of having the character of unavoidable actions to lessen the impact of the crisis. The militarization of the poorest sectors, the persistence of charitable models and the spectacularization of aid, today exacerbated pornographically, must be understood as the reproduction of a social structure configured several decades ago. We end up remembering the immense possibility that the emergency offers as a springboard for non-dependent social practices.

HUNGER, BODY AND EMOTION

Hunger is a social phenomenon that impacts the body. People need to feed to maintain the minimum state of reproduction of the organic processes that constitute what is called the body. The human person seen from a biological perspective is a complex interrelation between the volume of nutrients ingested, the energy expended to obtain them, and the quantum social energies available to manage these two components.

Hunger is a phenomenon of great variability that has various nuances: there is no single modality of hunger. Among the main types of hunger that can be identified in a diet, we find the following three: a) acute hunger, which is an intermittent phenomenon, with periodic but not continuous exacerbations and restitution; b) chronic hunger, of persistent and prolonged action, at the same time, that it can be qualitative or quantitative hunger - or both - depending on whether it refers to a diet with insufficient protein and vitamins or with insufficient calories; and finally, c) hidden hunger, which refers to malnutrition based on the lack of essential micronutrients for the biological, psychological and social development of people (De Castro, 1962). The three types of hunger coexist worldwide, locating themselves to a greater or lesser extent in some countries and spreading differentially across the social strata. Today, hidden hunger is found in both industrialized and poorer countries; in the former due to excess consumption, and in the latter due to the decrease or absence of certain foods, to which chronic hunger and acute hunger are added as part of the global reality. This points to hunger as a primarily social fact since "hidden hunger today constitutes the most typical form of human-made hunger" (De Castro, 1962, p.54). But what is relevant about hidden hunger or malnutrition is not only the lack of nutrients but its extension over time and the consequences it generates, since hunger will not only have consequences on the bodies of people who experience it. It will also impact their offspring and thus the entire process of social structuring. Taking this characterization elaborated by De Castro and placing it in the context of the body, we find a conceptualization proposal around hunger from a vision of the sociology of bodies/emotions that emphasizes their relational character. So, individual hunger refers to the "lack of nutrients" experienced by the individual body at the biological level (socially understood). It refers to the absence of nutrients (in a broad sense) for the reproduction of that body. It is enacted at the level of the relations between individuals, social organizations, and the environment. Subjective hunger affects the "auto-reflexivity of the self", i.e., it links the consequences of "identity" order, in the cognitive sphere which are related to hunger. It is enacted in the field of the relations of the human being with himself and its consequences in the embodied self-image of the subjects. Social hunger has an impact on the social presentation of the subject" (Scribano and Eynard, 2011, p.67).

Thus, we understand that individual hunger refers to the relationship between the human being and the environment, and subjective hunger refers to the relationship of the human being, while social hunger articulates the other two planes in connection with a life lived in a society. At the same time, these distinctions of hunger are connected with the distinctions of the body; therefore, hunger will affect the bodies on their individual, subjective and social[1] planes due to the unequal distribution of energy and nutrients, jeopardizing the corporeal existence as well as the possibility and power of action (Boragnio, 2018).

Bodies exist in connection with the environment from the processes that occur in the interaction between the brain, the central nervous system, nutrients and energies. Specifically, the concept 'body energy' refers to the direct relationship between the body and nutrients as a result of the exchange of physiological systems and biological processes that allow the durability of systemic functioning. This brings us closer to understanding the direct relationship that occurs between nutrients and the possibilities of action since social energy arises from this relationship, which "is based on body energy and refers to its distribution processes as a substrate of the conditions of movement and action. The power to plan, execute and resolve the consequences of the agents' actions constitutes the social energy that they have" (Scribano and De Sena, 2016, p.116).

While body energy is directly linked to nutrients, without nutrients there will be nobody energy, so the greater the nutritional deficiency, the less the possibility of action. At the same time, "social energies are closely related to bodily energies, since the greater the nutritional deficiency, the greater the probability of structuring a set of weak human relationships" (Scribano and De Sena, 2016, p.116). Therefore, the possibility and power to plan and execute the action will be conditioned by the availability of energy and, thus, by the possibility of access to food. For this reason, it must be taken into account that the availability of food resources alters the quantities and the energy qualities that each individual has at their disposal, allowing these bodies to reproduce and be socially available. Thus, hunger will configure in the bodies small potentialities of the possible states of life of the subjects as social agents. Meanwhile, unequal distribution and appropriation of energy and nutrition affect the corporal energies and, therefore, the social energies. This defines hunger as a central experience

---

[1] The individual body refers to phylogenetic logic, to the articulation between the organic and the environment; the subjective body is configured by self-reflection, in the sense of "I" as a centre of gravity through which multiple subjectivities are woven and passed, and the social body that is (in principle) the social made body. See Scribano, 2007; Scribano, 2005.

of life, as it is structuring of emotions and sensibilities. Hunger highlights the intersections and networks between bodies/emotions due to their socially constructed character, while the direct relationship between energies and nutrients establishes limits and socio-biological spaces from which it is possible to observe how the individual body is the result of policies of bodies and policies of emotions, and its consequences that organize the reproduction of bodies and their availability.

Poverty and Hunger in Pre-Pandemic Argentina

Hunger is always there. In Argentina, since the 1970s, poverty has continued to manifest itself as a problem of great magnitude and associated with it is the reproduction of forms of hunger. In the last quarter of the 20th century, there were global transformations that gave shape to what is known as the "new social question", the sociabilities and experiences of poverty and hunger being a fundamental part of the politics of sensibilities across the century. In Latin America and the Caribbean, the problems related to the resources necessary for the reproduction of life implied an approach and strategies for the regulation of conflict and social consensus. For the first decades of the 21st century, new poverty assistance interventions were required that would reach levels of great massiveness. For the year 2017, the number of people living in poverty reached 184 million, approximately 30.2% of the region's population, of which 62 million were in extreme poverty −10.2% of the population−, the highest percentage since 2008 (CEPAL, 2019).

In Argentina, poverty did not develop in a very different way. Poverty levels have skyrocketed since the early 1980s, with increases marked by economic crises, and it impacted between 20% and 35% of the population according to the period measured. At the same time, except for the 2001 political-economic crisis, poverty levels always found a new ceiling, higher than the previous measurement (De Sena, 2020). The latest data from the National Institute of Statistics and Censuses (INDEC) referring to

31 urban agglomerates, involving a population of 28,022,735 people,[2] indicate that, for the second half of 2019, the percentage of households below the poverty line (LP) reached 25.9%, which represents 35.5% of the population. Within this set, 8% of people (5.7% of households) can be distinguished below the indigence line (LI)[3] (INDEC, 2020).

Along with the historical journey that can be made through poverty data, data on social food policies must be added as ways of responding, regulating, normative, normalizing and mitigating conflict (Grassi, 2003; De Sena, 2011). Since the 1970s, the availability of food worldwide has been increasing. And since 1985 full availability of food was reached worldwide. This means that, statistically, with the current world food production, all the inhabitants of the world could obtain 2,700 Kilocalories (Kcal) daily[4] (Aguirre, 2010). However, for that year, the Food and Agriculture Organization of the United Nations (FAO) registered 875 million people as malnourished (Aguirre, 2015). Currently, the figure rises to 820 million people who suffer from chronic hunger and reaches almost 2 billion if we talk about those who suffer from hidden hunger and malnutrition (FAO, 2019). In this way, it is exposed that hunger is not a problem of availability or production, but rather a problem of access to food. In Argentina, in mid-1984, during the government of Raúl Alfonsín, the National Food Program (PAN)[5] was launched, which consisted of delivering food bags to families that presented some nutritional risk, popularly known as "box PAN". This was conceived as a two-year emergency program, but President Alfonsín kept it running until the end of his term. In the beginning, the PAN was estined for 907,360 families; in 1985, it was extended to 1,487,118, but three years later, boxes were being distributed to 1,506,470 families[6] (Sordini, 2018).

---

[2] The total population of Argentina estimated for 2020 is 45,376,763 people.

[3] This refers to the fact that below the poverty line is 2,423,562 households, that is, 9,936,711 people, of which 2,236,739 people are indigent. These data are constructed from the Permanent Household Survey, referring to 31 urban agglomerates. https://www.indec.gob.ar/uploads/informesdeprensa/eph_pobreza_02_195EFE752E31.pdf

[4] The amount of Kcal changed over time.

[5] 'PAN' is the acronym in Spanish.

[6] A separate issue is the number of boxes that were delivered, since although the number of families that were part of the PAN increased, the boxes did not always increase in the same

Subsequent governments, to date, have continued with food policy, but PAN was the first strictly food-related government program[7] and is considered the tracer thread of Argentine food programs, due to its scope, coverage and mode of implementation (Sordini, 2018). In this context, the "social question" was present, taking the form of hunger experienced by those social sectors that remained stuck in the place of the structural failure of the current accumulation regime. As De Sena maintains, "the processes of inequality and expulsion generated in the structuring of a society based on the commodification of life cause conflictive breaks that must be systematically remedied" (2014, p.155), and the taking of food is one of the main breaks that were configured from the 1980s.

Beginning in the 1990s, the Conditional Cash Transfer Programs (CCTP) began to be implemented as a modality of attention to poverty. These programs underwent rapid expansion and attained a massive reach, but at the same time that they were incorporated, those referring to food were not neglected, therefore the beginning of the overlap of programs can be observed. From 1990 to date, a variety of national food programs have been established. Among those that are still in force are the ProOrchards program, which has been operating since 1990, the Program for the Promotion of the Welfare of the Elderly (PPB), since 1992, and the National Plan for Food Security (PNSA), which was reconverted in 2003. To these, we can add the National Care Prices Program, which began in 2014.[8]

At present, the current food policy at the national level is called Plan Argentina contra el Hambre and "it is supported by the strengthening of the

---

proportion. Thus, we found that, if in 1987 16,488,304 boxes were delivered to 1,341,078 families, in 1988, 14,950,678 boxes were delivered for a little more than 165,000 extra families (Aguirre, 1990).

[7] In 1936, Law 12,341, "Palacios Law", was enacted, which was regulated in 1938. It attempted a "response from the State to the health, food and nutrition problems of the maternal and child population of Argentina, in a situation of poverty" (Abeya, 2016, p.591), but it was only put into national operation in 1952 delivering milk under the name of Maternal and Child Plan, which continues to this day.

[8] To this, it is necessary to add the Universal Assignment per Child (UAC) that was implemented in 2003 and the Pregnancy Allowance for Social Protection, since 2011. Both programs enter the conceptualization of PTCI since they grant money through transfer in exchange for some conditionalities. For more detail, see De Sena, 2011; Dettano, 2019.

actions carried out by the National Program for Food and Nutrition Security. It implies the promotion and strengthening of Access to the Basic Market Basket." (Argentina, n/d-b). Within this program, there is the Alimentar Card, which is a pre-loaded card that allows you to buy food – except for alcoholic beverages– and is intended for mothers or fathers with sons and daughters up to 6 years of age who receive the UAC, for pregnant women who from 3 months after pregnancy receive the Pregnancy Allowance, and people with disabilities who receive the Universal Assignment per Child. This program is "a comprehensive food supplement policy" (Anses.gob, n/d). As of March 11, 2020, 1,100,000 cards were delivered and "it is anticipated to deliver more than 1,500,000 cards, which will reach more than 2,800,000 recipients" (Argentina.gob.ar, 2020, March 16).

Hunger as a topic was of concern to various governments as well as serving as a political flag –and it is again today. This brief overview shows that, since the implementation of the PAN, the target population did not overcome the need for help to respond to their food needs. Thus, the applied programs, far from solving the food problem, denote a plot that sustained over time not only the dependence of the recipients on them and the reproduction of inequalities but also an increase in the number of people who are in need of state interventions. In this way, we can observe that, in Argentina, for a long time, there have been food policies that attest with their mere presence that hunger is always in any of the aforementioned modalities, thus configuring the pre-pandemic context of a structural problem: the uneven distribution of nutrients. In what follows we will describe the special association between militarization, policing, spectacularization and the commodification of aid that actions against hunger imply in the days of the COVID-19 Pandemic.

Hunger Interventions and Policies

In the context of the generalized crisis produced by the planetary extension of the COVID-19 pandemic, the Argentine National State designed a battery of state actions to avoid its untimely and deadly eruption. Since the beginning of the Preventive and Compulsory Isolation decreed by the National Government on March 20, a reinforcement of state assistance to the poorest families in the Metropolitan Area of Buenos Aires and the country in general began. The Army and the Churches are involved in a variety of them, at the same time as solidarity actions by companies were added, which had as a point of maximum visibility the holding of a televised event to raise funds for aid to the Red Cross.

Army, Food and Conflict

A basic feature of state interventions in this time of pandemic is the use of the war metaphor to describe the set of actions configured to lessen their impact. The President of the Nation in his speech announcing the Isolation maintained:

> "I thank you too, you are part of those who are exempt from the rule of staying at home, those who work in the media, journalists, I thank you very much for being here, I please ask that you help me to inform well, because as I told you last time, *one is fighting against an invisible enemy, who gets into our room, and one cannot detect it, but one has two fights: they are the fight against the pandemic and the fight that is constantly going on against psychosis*, those feeling that everything is very serious, that everything is irreparable and that nothing can be done." (Words from the President, 2020, March 20)

In this generalized and normalized context of the war metaphor, the participation of the Armed Forces is something very foreseeable as a material "reinforcement" of this war due to the politics of sensibilities launched by an invisible external enemy: biologically and psychologically invisible. In Argentina, the Army in the streets implies updating phantoms of the set of policies of the sensibilities associated with dictatorships. Although the presence and reconversion of the Gendarmerie to policing tasks has indeed become daily since at least 2004, the decision to "use" the army is a practice that fortunately has not been naturalized. The Argentine Army is currently forming part of the emergency plan about the pandemic. On its website it specifies:

> "In compliance with the directives issued by the national executive power, the Argentine Army enlists and prepares for the maintenance of the necessary means so that the Operational Command of the Joint Chiefs of Staff of the Armed Forces uses the necessary military resources (mainly health and logistics) to support the community in this Emergency caused by the COVID 19 Pandemic." (Argentina.gob.ar, 2020, March 27)

At the beginning of this fulfilment of tasks, they were involved with the logistical service of food distribution and food assistance. For example, in La Matanza,[9] Army personnel are deployed to carry out food distribution tasks –rice stew, noodle stew or lentil stew– in three-hour shifts per day, in which 24,000 food rations are distributed daily (Ayerdi, April 5, 2020). The explanation for the need to call upon the army to carry out this task focuses on the fact that "a food delivery operation of this magnitude is unprecedented" (Fuego Simondet, April 5, 2020) and that the army has the necessary resources such as kitchen equipment, industrial-size cooktops and the logistics necessary for the distribution.

These tasks gain greater visibility based on observing the geographical location map of military personnel, whose activities are detailed and range from assembling tents and beds for patient isolation, water supply, food processing and distribution, to satellite telecommunications support, air patrol and reconnaissance flights; these activities are concentrated in the east, northeast, west, northwest and the Metropolitan Area of Buenos Aires (Argentina.gob.ar, n/d-a).

But, the participation of the Army in the social tasks of the pandemic must be related to the diversity of "anti-looting" plans that are carried out mainly in the Metropolitan Area of Buenos Aires by the Security Forces. In this sense, an Emergency Operations Centre was created, made up of the

---

[9] It is the largest and most populous party in the Metropolitan area of Buenos Aires and in the province of Buenos Aires. It has a population of 1,775,816 inhabitants according to the 2010 census.

areas of Security, Social Development and Health (Ayerdi, April 5, 2020) to work together on an emergency plan linked to avoiding social conflict. This further complicates the Army's presence with the phantom structure of the looting associated with the 2001 crisis and the set of social responses to various food, poverty and work crises. In the recent history of Argentina, it is possible to verify, in the last four decades, the repetition of the crisis, looting and repression connection.

> "In this sense, the records of 'Nueva Mayoría' (2013) indicate that, for the period 1989 and 2013, 3,356 cases of looting have taken place, place in the context of the "outbreak of hyperinflation" (1989) some 676 cases; in the "outbreak of convertibility" (2001) 875 cases, 10 to which 151 lootings occurred in the first weeks of 2002 are added. In the subsequent period, looting has a low frequency (2003: 14 cases; 2008: 9 cases; 2009: 5 cases; 2010: 26 cases; 2011: 11 cases) until December 2012. That month, the looting began in Bariloche, spreading to several provinces, reaching a relative peak of 228 cases. In 2013, the phenomenon acquired a greater magnitude, accounting for a total of 1,266 cases (surpassing previous peaks)." (Scribano and Lisdero 2017, p. 338)

On April 15, the President of the Nation, Alberto Fernández, gave a speech at the Gendarmería School where he not only referred to the health/economy dichotomy but also announced the tripling of the Gendarmería's participation as a force that will control "compliance with quarantine" in La Matanza (Coronavirus en Argentina..., April 15, 2020). As of that day, the Gendarmerie is in charge of carrying out security care and quarantine control tasks in the largest municipality in the country (Fernando..., April 15, 2020). Given this, the communal chief ended the event saying that:

> "Today is a happy day for La Matanza. The President came to fulfil our request for more than four years: that the National Gendarmerie patrol the streets of La Matanza again. Today we are responding to a complaint from all our neighbours. That an institution so loved by our citizens returns to our streets generates a lot of tranquillity, because the Gendarmerie came to take care of the best capital we have, our people.

> (…) That the National Gendarmerie returns in these difficult times that we are living in Argentina and the world with the coronavirus pandemic, it also gives great peace to all the neighbours." (Fernando ..., April 15, 2020)

To this must be added that at the beginning of the period of Preventive and Compulsory Isolation there was an intense wave of control and "discipline" for those who broke the isolation, since "between March 21 and 31, only the national security forces had 644,009 people notified and/or controlled on public roads, of whom 19,939 were declared infringers" (Colectivo Editorial Crisis, April 1, 2020).

At the same time, in the future, there is already talk of a joint action initiative between state entities, social organizations, universities and the Army for the reconstruction of areas affected by the pandemic (Acción Social..., April 16, 2020).

To the deployment of the army in relation to food assistance has been added the aid of the national government. According to the journalistic note published on April 5 in the newspaper Perfil, the national government went from assisting eight million people to assisting 11 million. At the same time, "more than 300 million pesos was allocated to the municipalities for the purchase of food and there was an increase of 50% in the amount of aid to 3,000 soup kitchens that the ministry assists" (Ayerdi, April 5 2020). For their part, the municipal mayors signed agreements with supermarket chains, some of whom collaborate with the preparation of the food bags that the municipality distributes.

The National Administration indicates that the need for assistance increased as workers in the informal economy, who until now had no link with the ministry of social development, joined the demand for food. Additionally, there is an increase in attendance at soup kitchens, which look for a way to continue operating at a time when the demand from neighbours increases day by day. For this, they mainly make pot meals that allow the portions to be "stretched" to increase the quantity. Later, some soup kitchens organized a "delivery picketers" to bring food to the elderly in the neighbourhood. Likewise, the news highlights that, despite the changes and the efforts at organization, there was a lack of food (Colectivo Editorial Crisis, April 1, 2020) and that individual actions add to the attempts to feed neighbours and people in the neighbourhood (Cassini, April 18, 2020). This scene prepares us for the next section where it is possible to capture the unfolding of the commitment of all the Churches to addressing hunger in the context of COVID-19.

Churches and Charities

The history of the so-called "social question" has involved from its inception various forms of charity and philanthropy; the consequences of the pandemic bring with it new scenes of an elaborate narrative between good intentions, guilt, and manipulation.[10] For their part, the Churches organized an initiative called "#SeamosUno", in which various religious, Catholic, Christian and Jewish associations participate. They, in turn, solicited participation in the form of donations from associations and chambers of commerce. On its website, where "who we are" is defined, we see the slogan:

> "Together with CIAS-Compañía de Jesús, CARITAS, Banco de Alimentos, the Council of Evangelical Pastors of CABA, AMIA, ACIERA-Alianza Cristiana de Iglesias Evangelistas de la República Argentina and other business and social organizations, we have decided to launch the project #SeamosUno with to raise funds to be used to buy food and cleaning units, which will be distributed to those who need it most. The initiative implies an exhaustive control in the processes of collection, acquisition of products, assembly and control of boxes, delivery of the same. The project is being jointly audited by Deloitte, EY, KPMG and PWC to ensure the transparency of the process." (Seamosuno, 2020)

---

[10] We want to make clear, once again, that our criticism of being structural and sociological implies not making the mistake of adopting the ecological fallacy, that is attributing to each individual what in fact refers to the level of the collective and systemic.

It seeks to raise funds and donations in kind that allow the elaboration and distribution of food boxes (Ini, April 4, 2020). By April 17, 100,000 boxes with 15 kg of non-perishable food each had been distributed,[11] and funds are being raised to complete 400,000 more boxes, but the objective of the action is to deliver one million boxes of food to four million people, "especially to the informal sectors that do not have the habitual assistance of the State" (Naishtat, April 19, 2020).

In the conformation of these boxes, you can find donations from large national and some international companies, which provide products, boxes and logistics. The goal is to deliver 1,000,000 boxes. As we can see, the one million became a social fantasy: represented with the imaginary of multiplicity, of the exaggerated and the uncountable quantity of opulence.

The Jesuit priest Rodrigo Zarazaga, the main promoter of this practice, stated in an interview: "The people of the villages do not want chaos, but hunger leads to despair and their persistence can end in situations that we do not want; for this reason, this campaign seeks above all that no one goes hungry and that we stop in the face of the abyss" (Rubin, April 7, 2020). It is clear, once again, that the objective of conflict management and suppression of inequality lies in the conditions that preceded and pre-existed the pandemic. The other side of these commitments is the presence of the Army and its relationship with the Churches present in the poorest areas of the Metropolitan Area of Buenos Aires. In the GPS television program hosted by the journalist Rolando Graña, on A24,[12] on April 24, 2020, a segment titled: "Soup kitchens in the Metropolitan Area of Buenos Aires are seen. If there is no mass, there is a table". In this segment, the host of the program visits one of the Chapels of Padre Pepe[13] in the Barrio Independencia of the Partido de San Martin,[14] showing how, due to the

---

[11] The seamosuno page states: "Each box contains different food and hygiene products to cover the essential needs of a family for a week. Food products cover up to 56 food servings. Next, we give you the details of the products included: Rice/dry noodles - 4 kilos, Flour - 2 kilos, Tomato puree - 2 units, Tin cans - 2 units, Dried lentils or beans - 1 kg, Long-life milk - 3 litres, Mince can - 4 units, Canned fruits - 2 units, Toilet soap - 2 units, Detergent - 1 unit (300 cm3)" (Seamosuno, 2020).

[12] A news channel that can be seen throughout the country.

[13] Argentine priest dedicated to helping in the villas of the Metropolitan Area of Buenos Aires.

[14] The Metropolitan Area of Buenos Aires

prohibition of religious ceremonies and the food emergency, the chapel has become a community feeding centre. In the scene, lasting 1.36:33 minutes, you can see the host of the program showing how to eat where mass is commonly celebrated and showing the place to viewers, while saying: "[we can see that] the care of the Parish, the order… is in charge of army personnel… ",[15] while at the same moment, the camera takes a shot of two uniformed men and women, standing in a military posture. The synthesis is more than clear, the two institutions that guarantee social and moral order together in an intervention against hunger, the questions that arise are more than obvious: How will the situation of citizen security be if the Army has to guarantee order? What will be the level of poverty if it is the Church that must complement/replace the functions of the municipal state? The first answer, also obvious, is that this is Argentina before, during and after the Pandemic. One more band in Moebio's to which our investigation takes us here is the connection between dealing with hunger and the show.

Spectacle and Pandemic Sensibilities

The COVID-19 pandemic involves a contradictory set of modifications in sensitization policies on a planetary scale, and one of the most evident aspects is the acceleration of the spectacularization through the mass media and social networks. In Latin America, at least, every earthquake, volcano eruption, hurricane, torrential rain leaves bare what society only hides behind a pornographic acceptance: the existence of some structural absence.

With the "Teleton",[16] at the regional level, and with "A sun for children"[17] in Argentina, as paradigmatic television programs of the spectacularization of humanism diminished in its form of "anonymous donation", it constitutes one of the pillars of the systematic acceptance of the object of the collection: inequality about televised absence.

---

[15] https://www.youtube.com/watch?v=_CsFzAfOEUo
[16] https://teleton.org/
[17] https://es.wikipedia.org/wiki/Un_sol_para_los_chicos

The centrality of the show is one of the fundamental components of global awareness policies:

> "...the processes of crisis and metamorphosis of capitalism have been associated with staging and spectacularity. From the Paris Fair of 1910, through the Hitlerian concentration camps, to NASA's launches, capitalism has always shown its power through public spectacles. Today, in the Internet era and live broadcasts for billons of subjects, the spectacularization takes (and re-takes) other features to gain importance and centrality. All that is lived must be represented in public, massively transmitted and recognized/approved by "many". Every day of spectacle implies the appearance of a "reality show"-spirituality... ." (Scribano 2017, p. ...)

On April 5, the programme "United by Argentina" was broadcast, a television program organized at the request of the wife of President Alberto Fernández to the Argentine Red Cross to channel donations to acquire basic supplies for the pandemic: mouth cap, gel, respirators, etc. The program - which was broadcast in unison on all the broadcast channels and in which the collection of 88 million pesos was reached between donations and advertising guidelines (Trzenko and Fernández Cruz, April 5, 2020) - sought to "provide the opportunity Argentines to come together in the same voice of solidarity" (Unidos por Argentina [United for Argentina], n/d).

When closing the program (in a pre-recorded video of 3:56 minutes) Fabiola Yañez - first lady of the country - said "*...Thank you for being there ... I love you, love us, we love each other*."

The television special lasted almost 6 hours, in which recognized figures from the show and local television made their appearance, taught viewers recipes to cook at home, showed activities that could be shared with the family at home, and doctors known to the public advised about how to prevent and control coronavirus. At the same time, tributes were offered to the security forces, accompanied by speeches and the language of war. Thus, there was talk of "an invisible enemy", of a "silent war" and allusions were made to the Falklands War.[18]

Along with this special moment and demonstration of donation, it is also possible to find other initiatives by businessmen, unionists and officials around food and its distribution that are "made known" or that are directly part of the marketing of companies. An example is Orange Card, which targets its advertisements with the motivation "we can all do it together" and aims to donate 20,000,000 pesos.[19] As another example, in Chubut a fishing vessel that had to make a transfer trip caught 40 tons of hake (with fishermen who carried out the work as solidarity cooperation, not charging wages) to "distribute it among the poorest sectors of three cities in the province of Chubut " at Easter (Carpena, April 9, 2020).

All this has been complemented by numerous proposals for donations and contributions from a "solidarity of companies" of various kinds, amongst which stands out that of the "Group One Led", the leading firm in advertising business on Led screens:

> "With the focus on awareness, Miranda and his company decided to donate advertising space on their screens to help protect against the pandemic. How does it work? As he explained, it is a campaign that is projected free of charge on more than 60 screens located on public roads throughout the country where they transmit dynamic content in real-time that promote care and protection against COVID-19 and that are part of the "Stay Home" campaign." (Zanotti, April 8, 2020)

The need is to make the population and the newly connected advertising media known in a society where if you don't see you don't feel. Thus, shows, celebrities, companies, and advertising reconnect "as they know how to do it": the best way to generate an impact is by creating

---

[18] During those days, in various places on social networks, allusions were made to a historic and well-remembered program called "The 24 hours of the Falklands" which "... was a program broadcast in 1982 for 24 hours to raise funds for the men who were to fight the Falklands War. However, although the fate of the proceeds cannot be established, it is clear from the statements of its protagonists that it never reached its destination." https://es.wikipedia.org/wiki/Las_24_horas_de_las_Malvinas

[19] https://www.naranja.com/donaciones

sensibilities. Where there are no state resources, the spectacular sensibilities raised to serve as an appeal to dissolve institutional responsibility. Once again, Argentina's everyday reality appears in exceptional times.

HUNGER GAMES IN THE CONTEXT OF A PANDEMIC

In the movie "The Hunger Games",[20] games with the same name are developed, which are a televised competition for the hungry to survive.

> "The nation of Panem emerged from the ruins of what was once known as North America. 74 years ago, the 12 poverty-stricken districts in Panem revolted against the wealth that the Capitol controls. After its overwhelming victory, the Capitol devised "The Hunger Games." Each year, each district must hold a raffle (known as the harvest) to choose a man and a woman (ages 12-18) to participate in "The Hunger Games," a competition in that each of the 24 participants (known as tributes) will fight to the death in a televised arena until only one is alive. However, this is simply an annual reminder to the twelve districts of their authority and as punishment for the rebellion made 74 years ago."[21]

As in this film, the Argentine National State, in coordination with that of the Province of Buenos Aires, inaugurated an intervention based on the militarization of the struggle for survival. The "presence of the army" in the Metropolitan Area of Buenos Aires (and later throughout the country) and the results of containment are obvious: given the impossibility of quarantine by millions of people, the risk of social conflict increases and this leads to the pursuit of three goals: a) organize the population "on-the-street" (queues, clubs, neighbourhood centres, schools, etc.), b) reduce the risk of looting and c) control crime in the "assisted" areas.

---

[20] The Hunger Games is a science fiction, action and drama movie. Directed by Gary Ross and based on the best-selling novel of the same name by Suzanne Collins. It stars Jennifer Lawrence, Josh Hutcherson, Elizabeth Banks, Liam Hemsworth, and Woody Harrelson.

[21] https://es.wikipedia.org/wiki/Los_juegos_del_hambre_(pel%C3%ADcula)#Recepci%C3%B3n

These practices, beyond the obvious consequences for the risk of contagion, imply legitimization of the police and of the armed forces, the consolidation of the food dependency and the acceptance of the almost non-existent capacity of the Social Organizations which today occupy positions in the Ministry of Social Development among other state agencies.

The religions, with obvious and indisputable goodwill, reproduce a mechanism of direct assistance with the support of the technology of the 21st century - traceability of what is delivered - but with the charitable scheme of the 19th century where the other continues to be a passive agent and receiver. The articulation of different religious expressions, especially between the Christian and Catholic churches, guarantees the initiative a reticular procedure that efficiently links need and satisfaction, but with the limitation of the duration and contingency of such assistance.

The companies have initiated a set of interventions as we have narrated, but the "public-private television festival" is the one with the most massive consequences. Three elements should be highlighted: a) the open and massive television channels are the vehicles of the initiative, reproducing the political economy of current morality, conflating the logic of the show, donation and enjoyment; b) the reproduction of diminished humanism and the trivialization of the good; and c) the consecration of state failures in the acquisition of supplies necessary to face the health crisis.

To close the interpretation that we have been making, we want to point towards the recognition of two intervention devices on the survival of the poorest and hungry.

The s+c+c device (state+churches+companies) that was undoubtedly designed to "alleviate" the crisis, has an unintended consequence of its action and performative effectiveness: it clearly shows that Argentina was already in crisis. It shows that the depth of the crisis is such that there is nothing more appropriate than the word Emergency to describe it: the weak institutional fabric emerges. And the S+I+E (State + Intervention + Emotions) device, understood as an active equation in interventions on hunger, functions in terms of the policies of sensibilities that the construction of specific emotions provides in the context of the pandemic and food.

The diminished humanism that characterizes the aforementioned spectacularization is constituted by "a set of practices that operate as a mechanism for suturing differences and inequalities between classes. These practices are characterized, among other features, by inverting the place of the collective and the individual, erasing their differences; dilute social cooperation regimes, replaced by blaming fictions; leave the receiving subjects in an iterative situation as a grantee; replace state presence with private action; and re-inaugurate philanthropy and private charity as mechanisms for attention to deficiencies" (Scribano 2014, p. 81).

Beyond the analysis provided here, and further, on what emerges when the crisis deepens, beyond the politics of perversion (Scribano, 2015) and further than meanness and selfishness, it is possible to perceive hundreds of thousands of interstitial practices that speak of a different way of understanding what is happening. Precisely, the fact that millions of people around the world and in Argentina have grasped the "logic of what emerges" implies that there are other opportunities not to repeat the spectacular militarization of a diminished humanism that always leaves us in a state of dependency.

References

Acción social y voluntaria: el plan que pretende ser el nuevo "Operativo Dorrego". (16 de abril de 2020). [Social and Voluntary Action: the new Dorrego Operation] *Perfil.* Recovered from https://m.perfil.com/noticias/politica/accion-social-voluntaria-generacion-patriotica-ministerios-universidades.phtml?rd=1

Abeya Gilardon, E. (2016) Una evaluación crítica de los programas alimentarios en Argentina, *Salud Colectiva*, 2016, 12(4), Universidad Nacional de Lanús. pp. 589-604, DOI: 10.18294/sc.2016.935. [A critical assessment to the food programs in Argentina, *Collective Health*, 2016, 12 (4), National University of Lanús].

Aguirre, P. (2015). *La situación mundial.* En P. Aguirre, D. Díaz Córdova, & G. Polischer (Eds.), *Cocinar y Comer en Argentina Hoy* (pp. 23-32). Buenos Aires, Argentina: Sociedad Argentina de Pediatría. [*The world situation*. In P. Aguirre, D. Díaz Córdova, & G. Polischer (Eds.), *Cook and Eat in Argentina Today* (pp. 23-32). Buenos Aires, Argentina: Argentine Society of Pediatrics.].

Aguirre, P (2010) *La comida en los tiempos del ajuste.* En: Susana Torrado (dir.) *El costo social del ajuste (Argentina 1976-2002).* [*The Food in times of Crisis.* In: Susana Torrado (dir.) *The social cost of adjustment (Argentina 1976-2002)*]. Buenos Aires: Edhasa.

Aguirre, P. (1990). *El Pan "Programa alimentario nacional" Informe sobre su implementación entre los años 1984-1990.* Buenos Aires. [Documento Técnico Inédito] [*The NFP "National Food Program" Report on its implementation between 1984-1990.* Buenos Aires. (Unpublished Technical Document)]

Anses.gob (s/f) Tarjeta Alimentar: *Anses.* https://www.anses.gob.ar/tramite/tarjeta-alimentar

Argentina.gob.ar (2020, 16 marzo) L*a tarjeta Alimentar se entregará por Correo Argentino*. [*The Alimentar card will be delivered by Correo Argentino.*] https://www.argentina.gob.ar/noticias/la-tarjeta-alimentar-se-entregara-por-correo-argentino

Argentina.gob.ar (2020, 27 de marzo) El Ejército Argentino se alista para la Emergencia. [The Argentine Army is getting ready for the Emergency]. *Argentina.gob.ar/ejercito.* https://storymaps.arcgis.com/stories/b99a11f351d9481387e51e6393a11b62

Argentina.gob.ar (n/d-a) El Ejército y el COVID-19. El Ejército Argentino en todo el país. [The Army and COVID-19. The Argentine Army throughout the country]. *Argentina.gob.ar/ejercito.* https://www.argentina.gob.ar/ejercito/covid-19

Argentina (n/d-b) Argentina contra el hambre. Hacia un país con soberanía y seguridad alimentaria: *Argentina.gob.ar.* [Argentina (n/d) Argentina against hunger. Towards a country with food sovereignty and security: *Argentina.gob.ar.*] Retrieved from https://www.argentina.gob.ar/argentinacontraelhambre

Ayerdi, Rosario (5 de abril de 2020) Emergencia social: despliegan el plan "antisaqueo" en el conurbano bonaerense. [Social emergency: they deploy the "anti-looting" plan in the Buenos Aires suburbs.] *Perfil.* Retrieved from https://www.perfil.com/noticias/politica/en-el-conurbano-despliegan-el-plan-antisaqueo.phtml

Boragnio, A. (2018) Disposable commensality: strategies for the selection of meals in the office. *Eureka: Social and Humanities.* N°5 (2018). ISSN: 2504-5571. pp. 16-28.

Cassini, Á. (18 de abril de 2020) Coronavirus en La Matanza: todas las noches los vecinos hacen cola en la puerta de su casa y ella les da de comer [Coronavirus in La Matanza: all the nights waiting for food while she serves the dinner]. *Clarín.* Retrieved from https://www.clarin.com/zonales/
coronavirus-isidro-casanova todas-noches-vecinos-hacen-cola-puerta-casa-da-comer_0_d8wNRzd3C.html

Carpena, R. (9 de abril de 2020) Un "buque solidario" pescó 40 toneladas de merluza para los sectores pobres de Chubut. [A supportive Vessel: four tons of hake were caught for poorer sectors of Chubut Province]. *Infobae.* Recovered from https://www.infobae.com/politica/ 2020/04/09/un-buque-solidario-pesco-40-toneladas-de-merluza-para-los-sectores-pobres-de-chubut/

CEPAL (2019) *Panorama Social de América Latina 2018.* [*Social Program of Latin America 2018*]. ISBN: 9789211220087. Available at https://www.cepal.org/es/publicaciones/44395-panorama-social-america-latina-2018

Colectivo Editorial Crisis (1 de abril de 2020) informe sobre la cuarentena en los barrios populares. [Report on the effects of Lockdown in neighborhood]. *Crisis.* Recovered from https://revistacrisis.com.ar/notas/informe-sobre-la-cuarentena-en-los-barrios-populares?fbclid=IwAR2AzKPFVrQAiWhCmsilhLKaw-P73qaNplUi2mrflfB0WfJT9gTjoECe8y8

Coronavirus en Argentina: "Que nadie piense que por cuidar la salud uno está descuidando el futuro" afirmó Alberto Fernández. (15 de abril de 2020). [Coronavirus in Argentina: "Let no one think that by taking care of one's health one is neglecting the future," said Alberto Fernández]. *Clarín.* Retrieved from https://www.clarin.com/politica/coronavirus-argentina-nadie-piense-cuidar-salud-descuidando-futuro-afirmo-alberto-fernandez_0_21VVtAMZ6.html

De Castro, J. (1962) *Geopolítica del hambre. Ensayo sobre los problemas alimentarios y demográficos del mundo* [The Geopolitics of Hunger: essay review on the food and demographic problems worldwide]. Buenos Aires: Solar Hachette.

De Sena, A. (2020) *Pobreza y programas sociales en la Argentina de las últimas décadas.* En De Sena (comp) *Vulnerabilidad, pobreza y políticas sociales: abanico de sentidos América Latina, Europa y China.* (En prensa) [*Poverty and Wellness Programs in the Recent Decades*. In De Sena (comp.) *Vulnerability, Poverty and Social Policies: the broad range of senses in Latin America, Europe and China*. (In press)]

De Sena, A. (2014) *Las políticas hecha cuerpo y lo social devenido emoción: lecturas sociológicas de las políticas sociales.* [The emboded politics and the derivation of emotionalities: sociological readings]. Buenos Aires: Estudios Sociológicos Editora/Universitas. Avaiable in: http://estudiosociologicos.org/portal/lecturas-sociologicas-de-las-politicas/

De Sena, A. (2011) Promoción de micro-emprendimientos y políticas sociales: ¿Universalidad, focalización o masividad?, una discusión no acabada. [The rise of Micro-enterprises and social policies: Universality, Focalization or massification?, an unresolved discussion]. *Revista Pensamiento Plural,* 8(1), 5-36.

FAO (2019). El hambre en el mundo lleva tres años sin disminuir y la obesidad sigue creciendo [The Unresolved levels of hunger in the world after years of irresolution, while the obesity is still rising]. *Organización de las Naciones Unidas para la Alimentación y la Agricultura.* http://www.fao.org/news/story/es/item/1201670/icode/

Fernando Espinoza: "La Gendarmería volvió a La Matanza para cuidar a nuestra gente". (15 de abril de 2020). [Fernando Espinoza: "The Gendarmerie returned to La Matanza to take care of our people."]. *Infobae.* Recovered from https://www.infobae.com/politica/ 2020/04/ 16/fernando-espinoza-la-gendarmeria-volvio-a-la-matanza-para-cuidar-a-nuestra-gente/

Fuego Simondet, J. (5 de abril de 2020) El Ejército en La Matanza: una ayuda social al filo del abismo [The Army forces in Matanza: a double-edged sword]. *La Nación.* Retrieved from https://www.lanacion.com.ar/politica/el-ejercito-en-la-matanza-una-ayuda-social-al-filo-del-abismo-nid2350913

Grassi, E. (2003) *Políticas de Asistencia Focalizadas en el Desempleo y la Pobreza.* [Social Programs with focus on Unemployment and Poverty]. In *Políticas y problemas sociales en la sociedad neoliberal. La otra década infame (I) [Problems and inconsistencies of neoliberal society: Another Dreadful Decade (I)].* Buenos Aires: Espacio Editorial, pp. 221-302.

INDEC (2020) *Incidencia de la pobreza y la indigencia en 31 aglomerados urbanos. Segundo semestre de 2019*. En: *Condiciones de vida,* [*Poverty and Pauperism in the 31 Urban agglomerations.* In: *Life conditions*], Vol. 4, N°4. ISSN 2545-6660. https://www.indec.gob.ar/ uploads/informesdeprensa/eph_pobreza_02_195EFE752E31.pdf

Ini, C. (4 de abril de 2020) Coronavirus: la colecta Seamos Uno prepara las primeras 100.000 cajas de alimentos para distribuir. [Coronavirus: the campaign we are only one] *La Nación.* Retrieved from https://www.lanacion.com.ar/politica/coronavirus-comenzo-logistica-iniciativa-solidaria-seamos-uno-nid2350815

Naishtat, S (19 de abril de 2020) "Morfi o vendrán los saqueos", el pedido que disparó la asistencia. [Food or the new Lootings: the claim for social assistance.] *Clarín.* Recovered from https://www.clarin.com/ economia/economia/-morfi-vendran-saqueos-pedido-disparo-asistencia_0_edbjkoiJt.html

Rubin, S. (07 de abril de 2020) Rodrigo Zarazaga sj: "La gente de las villas no quiere el caos, pero el hambre lleva a la desesperación" [Slum-Dwellers do not want chaos: but hunger very well leads to desesperation] *Religión Digital.* https://www.religiondigital.org/america/Rodrigo-Zarazaga-jesuita-villas-desesperacion-hambre-coronavirus-campana-solidaria-seamos-uno_0_2220377966.html

Seamosuno (2020) Quienes somos: *#SeamosUno.* [Who we are: #Let'sbeOne.] https://www.seamosuno.com.ar/quienes-somos

Scribano, A. (2017) *Normalization, Enjoyment and Bodies/Emotions: Argentine Sensibilities.* New York: Nova Science Publishers, Inc.

Scribano, A. (2015b) *Una aproximación al estado de las sensibilidades en Argentina desde la(s) Politica(s) de la Perversión.* En: Rafael Sánchez Aguirre (Comp.) *Sentidos y sensibilidades: exploraciones sociológicas sobre cuerpos/emociones.* [*An approach to the state of sensibilities in Argentina from the Politic(s) of Perversion.* In: Rafael Sánchez Aguirre (Comp.) *Senses and sensibilities: sociological explorations on bodies/emotions.*] Buenos Aires: ES Editora, pp. 141-161.

Scribano, A. (2014) El don: entre las practicas intersticiales y el solidarismo. *Sociologias,* [The Gift: intersectial practices and reciprocity]. Porto Alegre, Universidade Federal do Rio Grande do Sul. Instituto de Filosofía e Ciencias Humanas. Programa de Pós-Graduaçao em Sociologia Porto Alegre. ISBN 1517 - 45221, Brasil, ano 16, no 36, mai/ago p. 74-103.

Scribano, A. (2007) *La sociedad hecha callo: conflictividad, dolor social y regulación de las sensaciones.* En Scribano, A. (comp.) *Mapeando interiores. Cuerpo, conflicto y sensaciones* [*Society comes into pieces: conflict, social pain and regulation of emotionalities.* In: Scribano, A. (Comp.) *Mapping the inner-worlds: body, conflict and sensations*]. Córdoba: Jorge Sarmiento Editor.

Scribano, A. (2005). *Geometría del conflicto: Estudios sobre acción colectiva y conflicto social.* [*Geomtry of Conflict: Social Action Studies and Social Conflict*]. Córdoba: Universitas.

Scribano, A. y De Sena, A. (2016) *Cuerpos débiles: energías, políticas alimentarias y depredación de bienes comunes.* En: Martins, P. & de Araújo Silva, M. (Org.) *Democracia, Pós-desenvolvimiento e gestão de benscomus. Perspectivas da América Latina e do Caribe.* [*Vulnerable Bodies: energies, Food Politics and Enviromental Predation.* In: Martins, P. & de Araújo Silva, M. (Org.) Democracy, Post-development and management of benscomus. Prospects for Latin America and the Caribbean.] Brasil: Editora. pp. 115-128.

Scribano, A. & Eynard, M. (2011) Sociologando: Hambre individual, subjetivo y social (reflexiones alrededor de las aristas límite del cuerpo). [Speaking of Sociology: hunger, subject and society]. *Boletín Científico Sapiens. Research Sapiens Research* Vol. 1 (2)-2011, pp: 65-69.

Scribano, A. & Lisdero, P. (2017). Saqueos en la Argentina: algunas pistas para su comprensión a partir de los episodios de Córdoba - 2013. [Lootings in Argentina: some hints to understand the lootings in Cordoba, 2013]. *Caderno CRH,* 30(80), 333-351. https://dx.doi.org/10. 1590/s0103-49792017000200008

Sordini, V. (2018) Nació con un PAN bajo el brazo! La transición a la democracia: entre el derecho y el subsidio a la alimentación, [The Lord gives children the mean to feed them!: Transitional democracy: between the Right and the right to Food] *Unidad Sociológica I Número 12, Año 3* I, *febrero 2018-mayo 2018* I *Buenos Aires.*

Trzenko, N. y Fernández Cruz, M. (5 de abril de 2020) Unidos por Argentina: se recaudaron cerca de 88 millones de pesos. [All united for Argentina: about 88 million pesos were collected.] *La Nación.* Recovered from https://www.lanacion.com.ar/espectaculos/ television/ como-sera-especial-unidos-argentina-transmision-simultanea-nid2350444

Unidos por Argentina (s/f) *TV Pública.* [United for Argentina (n/d) *Public TV.*] https://www.tvpublica.com.ar/programa/unidos-por-argentina/

Words from the President (2020, 20 de marzo) Palabras del presidente de la Nación, Alberto Fernández, luego de su reunión con los Gobernadores, para analizar la pandemia del coronavirus, COVID-19, desde Olivos: *Casa Rosada Presidencia.* https://www.casarosada.gob.ar/informacion/discursos/46783-palabras-del-presidente-de-la-nacion-alberto-fernandez-luego-de-su-reunion-con-los-gobernadores-para-analizar-la-pandemia-del-coronavirus-covid-19-desde-olivos

Zanotti, G. (8 de abril de 2020) Empresas activan campañas de donaciones para luchar contra el COVID-19. [Companies activate donation campaigns to fight COVID-19.] *Ámbit.com.* Recovered from https://www.ambito.com/negocios/pandemia/empresas-activan-campanas-donaciones-luchar-contra-el-covid-19-n5094167

In: Emotionality of COVID-19 ISBN: 978-1-53619-534-7
Editors: M. Korstanje and S. Adrian © 2021 Nova Science Publishers, Inc.

Chapter 3

The Enemy Inside

Primavera Fisogni*
La Provincia di Como, Italy

Abstract

The global world has recently been under attack from a new enemy, whose microscopic shape shuttered every aspect of human life: health, relations, social and economic frames. The COVID-19 outbreak can be compared to a war, with relation to the number of victims made worldwide. Still unknown in its several biological aspects, Coronavirus is currently going to update the concept of enemy. As I intend to argue, the pandemic brought to the forefront the idea of *enemy as an insider which* constantly *interacts with the host*. The enemy can be attacked only assuming it, making it part of both the individual body and the social body. According to this perspective immunization cannot be seen in terms of an exemption but properly as an inclusion. My reasoning starts from a short account of the classic paradigm of friend/enemy sketched by Schmitt (1932) and developed by Vitale (1992) in order to show the novelty of the 'enemy inside.' Then I'll take in consideration the processes that give rise to immunization, through the lens of General System Thinking (Urbani Ulivi, 2019) that better fit the purpose to

* Corresponding Author's E-mail: pfisogni@gmail.com.

explore such a complex topic. I'll reach the conclusion that immunization makes the enemy (virus) and the host (the biological substratum) adversaries: this dynamic, by reducing the dangerous potential of enemy, puts it under control. Thus, any process of immunization can be interpreted as the making of a community, differently from Esposito's theory (1998; 2001) of a sharp distinction between *immunitas* and *communitas* (immunity/community).

Keywords: coronavirus, enemy, conflict, immunization, immunity, community

UNDER ATTACK OF A VIRAL ENEMY[1]

An epidemic plague initially focused on China, affected the word as never before in the last century. A short account of it is necessary before investigating the topic of the present paper. The Coronavirus Disease 19 (COVID-19) outbreak has brought about a radical turn of the social, economic, and cultural scenario since January 2020. The speed of the contagion has spread faster than the SARS epidemic rush in 2009 so that the Chinese Government decided to lock down Wuhan, the main town of the Hubei region. Although the report from China profiled a red alert from the very beginning of the epidemic emergency, it took time before the WHO (World Health Organization) declared that the epidemic outbreak was turning into a global pandemic. Face masks, gloves, special protection and careful attention to cleaning have become new social practices for everybody. After struggling against the viral attack, the world is aware that the war is far from over and a new enemy is taking the scene. The micro-organism that affects all social levels in a macroscopic way is a case study also for philosophy and political sciences because it updates, with the power of an earthquake, models and frames that, after the pandemic, seem worn and inadequate.

---

[1] This investigation is dedicated to Mario Antonio Clerici, with whom I discussed the main argumentations of the present work.

The Virus as an Enemy: Limits of the Discourse

Since the very beginning, the Coronavirus pandemic has been equated by the media to a "public enemy number one" (Boseley, 2020), whose potential could be easily compared with that of terrorism, as the director-general of the World Health Organization Tedros Adhanom Ghebreyesus warned ("Viruses can have more powerful consequences than any terrorist action"). The media coverage focused on military metaphors for sketching its profile, so that COVID-19 was said to be the "biggest challenge since Second World War" (Angela Merkel, The Telegraph, 2020), "the invisible enemy" (James McAvoy, Daily Mail, 2020) who "moves among us unseen" (The Conversation, 2020) in the "frontline" (The Guardian).

The microscopic bio-organism is a veritable enemy for life because it moves inside blood circulation and the respiratory system. Differently from a parasite, which can be taken together as a companion, the virus immediately shows its hostile intentions to the guest, through a huge attack to the very heart of the life in itself. What makes the situation more complicated for COVID-19 is that, in the majority of the cases, the virus does not show itself with the unfriendly consequences of its deadly potential. As always happens for the phenomena described through metaphors, the war against COVID-19 highlights the limits of any discourse and the urgent need to know what sort of enemy coronavirus is. The conceptual difficulty that coronavirus designates does not only depend on the still unknown biological dynamics of the virus; as I intend to argue in my paper, the pandemic updated the notion of the enemy by introducing a substantial novelty within the traditional debate about this topic. More precisely, the pandemic provides us with a better understanding of how the concept of enemy works within the frame of the immunization processes, as will be explained in the following paragraphs.

Deeply interwoven with interdisciplinary implications, the term enemy is generally referred to an individual of whom to beware because of its dangerous potential. The notion of the enemy makes primarily refers to the opposite of friend, as someone we can trust and deal with. On the psychological ground, an enemy is a subject who gives rise to a cluster of bad feelings – fear, anxiety, anguish, terror – which are expected to destabilize a single individual (Gosio, 2020) or a community (Ceri and Lorini, 2019; Schlee, 2010). In his pioneering investigation on the concept of the enemy, the *Der Begriff des Politischen* (1932), Schmitt assumes that it is the intensity of the degree of association/dissociation to decide who is 'friend' (*Freund*) or 'enemy' (*Feind*) in political terms.

A very complex word, the enemy is rooted in the Latin word *inimicus*, formed by the negative element *in-*; hence, an enemy is "what a friend is not." In Slavic languages, where the enemy is *neprijatelj,* this conceptual framework is still relevant, different from the Latin and German languages, as noted by Vitale (1992). Schmitt shed light on the 'private enemy,' a concept that differs from the 'public enemy' (*Feind*) and the 'other/stranger' (*Fremde*). The best reference for framing a 'private enemy' can be found in the Latin word *hostis [host]*, an ambiguous term where two semantic areas are deeply intertwined: the one belonging to the guest as someone who is accepted, included, recognized and another one dealing with the enemy, who gives rise to hostile behaviors against the community (Plumper and Neumayer, 2010).

What makes an enemy a 'private foe'? The conceptual field of *hostis* embraces the main idea, among others, which deals with the domestic frame in which both the guest and the host are dwelling. It may be concluded that the ambiguity that entails the term is strictly related to the kind of relationship existing between two subjects, both within a commonplace. Despite the rough description, this passage is highly relevant in the perspective of this current investigation, because it could be applied to the immunization process, in order to prove that COVID-19 brought in to act a private enemy, a contemporary *hostis* who currently inhabits the global fears.

What Kind of Enemy? The Identification of the Foe

Only the identification of the enemy makes the hostile individual a target against whom to act, with good chances of stopping it. As Aho underlines, groups socially construct enemies according to five steps, moving from the naming of the foe, the most crucial rank of the operation followed by legitimation, mythmaking, sedimentation and ritual (Aho, 2010). Profiling the enemy in the process, often questioned (Lyon, 2003, 2007), through which the 'public enemy' is set up. It is proper at this point of the process that the traditional distinction between 1) enemy and 2) friend makes sense. When the foe is detachable, community glues together against it and empowers itself (Schlee, 2010). This dynamic, on which the classical idea of war is based, has been completely surpassed in the last two decades by global conflicts and especially by the war on terrorism, where the difficulty to focus on a visible enemy gave rise to the new categories of the 'terrorists from next door' and the 'lone wolves' (Fisogni, 2014, 2019).

In the struggle against a pandemic, as in any conflict, the need to focus on the public foe is necessary to delete it. When scientific investigations proved unable to forge biochemical weapons to flatten it, superstition and rage easily took their place. During the bubonic plague that struck Milan, in Italy, in 1630, the plague spreaders (the *untori*) were hunted and executed. These persons, as Italian leading novelist Alessandro Manzoni reported in the *Infamous Column* (La storia della Colonna infame, 1843), were innocent but reputed guilty by the crowd. The necessity of identifying them as 'public enemies' by the social community and the execution that occurred on the public square, was endorsed by the Milanese judges although it was illegal (Ciacca, 1985). As this episode witnesses, the wish to shape the enemy goes along with the necessity to bring a scapegoat onto the stage.

According to the victimization hypothesis theorized by Girard (1982), even if an innocent is going to be executed, the act is expected to solve a social crisis through exceptional measures that surpass any prescribed laws.

The COVID-19 pandemic updated this frame more softly. The single scapegoat, which is identified and then destroyed by the enemy, has been replaced by the collective ritual of wearing a face mask. Behind a behaviour due to the collective wealth, a powerful metaphorical operation for targeting the enemy can be noticed. In a pandemic, everyone can be seen as a potential enemy and a virus spreader. At the same time, anybody may be a victim of the virus itself. The two grounds of the phenomenon interfere, interact and are faced up together. As it happens with someone guilty for having committed a crime, in the lockdown as well as in the quarantine people have been imprisoned at home for weeks and have to abdicate several freedoms guaranteed by civil laws (Campi, 2020). We all were protected, we all had to guard against the enemy from the next door.

In the bubonic plague of 1630 ordinary justice was left outside tribunals, as Manzoni underlined, for allowing the public rage to compensate the frustration of coping with an epidemic that took nearly 50% of Milan's population. Although the constitutional laws of democratic countries consider several freedoms as unquestionable, social or pandemic emergencies, as happened within the Coronavirus outbreak, it nevertheless tends to inhibit several personal rights for the sake of public health. The lockdown experienced worldwide made it visible on a global scale. We are now in the condition to move into a further stage that will allow us to highlight the main novelty of the concept of enemy provided by the COVID-19. As I intend to argue, the pandemic brought on the scene the idea of the enemy as an insider. The enemy can be attacked by only assuming it, making it part of both the individual body and the social body. Hence, the topic of immunization becomes very key to reshaping this issue.

Immunization as the Integration between Host and Enemy

Immunization is a recurrent topic within the Coronavirus pandemic. In the biomedical language, it is the process that brings immunity or protection to the living organism. This kind of response, which is the specific reaction of the immune system to a pathogen, allows the system to generate an immunological memory that keeps the individual safe from the risk of getting infected by the same virus or bacteria. The second relevant process related to the immune system is its innate response to pathogenic attacks, by the immediate mobilization of cells against infection.

The origin of immunology as a science dates the inoculation of cowpox introduced by Jenner against smallpox in 1796; however, it should be ascribed to Pasteur the idea of inducing immunity throughout attenuated microorganism (vaccination) in 1880.

Mainly regarded as "a complex mechanism of integration of microbes into the cell community of the host" (Igea, 2015: 55), the term immunity is frequently applied to several different fields. During the last two decades, the concept expanded from the biological domain into political philosophy giving rise to a new field of investigations, especially in Italy where Esposito theorized (1998, 2001) immunity as the paradigm for globalization. In his analysis, immunity and community share the idea of an obligation, a *munus* in Latin, on which a couple of terms is semantically rooted. The immune person is someone who got free from the obligation and, for it, has temporary or placed himself outside the community. Although immunity is expected to safeguard the individual/social body, Esposito argues that it is at the same time something that inhibits the development of a community and, over a certain degree, it can destroy social cohesion.

As Igea argued from the biological perspective, there is a gap between "what 'immunity' etymologically means and what the term implies today" (2015: 55), however, the conceptual core of the word maintained certain stability throughout its semantic changes: it refers to an exemption/freedom of duties for some individuals with which other subjects have to comply. It is in fact in virtue of this particular condition, within the social/political discourse, that the social *community often looks at the immune as an outsider*, someone about whom to be cautious for his being out, free from a collective *munus*. Within the frame of the COVID-19 pandemic, an immune individual is someone free from the infectious disease, nevertheless, he remains involved at large with the hostile agent for having hosted it. The infection has changed his biological structure and made of him the 'other,' that's to say a subject that stands apart from the community and can be included only with a watchful approach.

At this point in the paper, a question arises. *Why does a community tend to isolate immune subjects?* They felt as potentially hostile as if they were still in relation with the pathogenic agent. I call this condition 'the enemy inside.' In the next paragraph, I'll seek to get deeper into this insight through the lens of General System Thinking.

Processes of Immunization: from Exemption to Integration

In this section, I aim to clarify the concept of the 'enemy inside,' as a result of the immunization process. This conceptual frame cannot be understood according to linear thinking because, as already seen in Esposito's theory, immunity and community stand apart as separate poles. Therefore, I suggest changing the interpretative paradigm, by investigating this topic through the lens of General System Thinking (Urbani Ulivi, 2019; Minati and Pessa, 2019).

According to GST, living phenomena are considered in term of open systems; it means that they are not mere aggregations or sums of parts, but primarily dynamic units, to which belong qualities that depend upon many interactions and processes, internal or external to the system, the continuous exchange with the environment that gives rise to systemic properties or II type systemic properties. According to this philosophical perspective, immunization cannot be considered first and foremost an isolated phenomenon which stands outside a community. Living systems, as human individuals or societies, are coherent structures engaged in "a continual (extended) critical transition" (Minati, 2019: 16). This instability is due to the degree of organization that is "maintained by the integration/regulation activities of the organism that is by its global coherent structure."

It follows that immunization is a twofold shaped phenomenon: it is a dynamic system involved in a permanent critical transition. If we come back to Esposito's dualistic frame (1998, 2001), it becomes clearer why the immune subject cannot be fully integrated by the community. An immune is someone who experienced a radical change in the very intimate texture of the system. Thus, he can change his mind, he can assume behaviors and beliefs that are different from the ones shared by the social group and, for it, they may destabilize society in reason of his 'permanent critical transition.' Communitas of non-immune people, on the contrary, maintains its properties stable over time, "including evolutionary patterns" (Minati, 2019: 16). A community tends to glue together its components, leaving outside whatever can destabilize it, within an incessant demand of self-protection. However, being involved in several processes, a community needs preventive immunization from any thrust that might undermine its coherence.

The contradiction that *immunitas/communitas* paradigm brings to surface can be easily solved, within the frame of General System Thinking, by taking in account the conflict between 1) transition and 2) coherence of change and stability, two aspects that are deeply intertwined in open systems that pertain to life's domain.

At this point in the discussion, we can take another step into the discussion.

Immune people and non-immune individuals can be equated to systems with different dynamics, which constantly interact. They show different degrees of reactivity to the thrust of the environment. Immunization belongs to the domain of dissipative structures, referring to the coexistence of change and stability (Prigogine, 1967, 1981, 1999). As Minati notes, non-equilibrium conditions allow the emergence of ordered structure. Furthermore, the stability of dissipative structures "is due to their ability to transfer a large amount of entropy to their environment" (Minati, 2019: 33). Concerning a community system, where stability is provided primarily by coherence, an immunization system constantly transfers energy outside itself, it is more dynamic and for it, less predictable. At this point, we can better grasp why immune subjects are perceived as destabilizing although immunity is a necessary step for protecting a social group: their access to the community brings into it the sphere of what is *out* and can be hostile *in* a community because it is not known.

In the next paragraph, we'll focus on these two poles.

In and Out, two Conflicting Poles?

The terms *in* and *out*, which take a relevant part in the friend/enemy discourse also belongs to the immunization process and, at large, to the dissipative systems, to which also immunization belongs. This consideration is highly relevant in order to move from the biological frame into the political environment. Before discussing this passage, I briefly recall that a *community* is the typical in-group society, where the individual share common values, laws, habits, cultures and way of life. The notion of humanity itself "can be understood as a set of concepts related by family resemblances" (M. Bilewicz, A. Bilewicz, 2012: 341). If commonalities are expected to paste together a society, they need to be constantly reinforced by differences which belong to the 'out' environment. The out-group is perceived as stranger, different, hostile. Qualities that properly belong to the semantic field of 'enemy,' as also Schmitt underlined in *Der Begriff des Politischen*, by assuming that *Fremde*" was primarily the other, the stranger" (Vitale, 1992: 92, translation is mine). The divide between the two poles is sharp in social dynamics, however in terms of open system processes, the two poles are closely involved in relation, in a continually in-out-in-out interaction.

In the dissipative systems – where change and stability coexist as seen before – the environment is a perfect copy of the system because of the interacting fluxes that move from both. It is the case, for example, of human brain dynamics, where environment is generally called 'the double' of the brain (Vitiello, 2010: 115). The entrance/exit streams have to balance to allow the stability of their interrelation. If the problem of enemy is considered from this perspective through the lens of General System Thinking, the terms *in/out* can hardly be separated. They are activities whose interaction is needed for allowing coherence. What makes it difficult for the community to include immunity and the related phenomena within its borders is the possibility to cope with processes that may bring about changes in the social environment. From the GST perspective, this is the particular kind of interactions that belong to any dissipative system. A community tends to prefer compatibility to irregularity or unpredictability. When the interaction is provided by dissipative systems like immunization, where the poles in/out are in constant relation, the possibilities that new emergences emerge is highly predictable. In terms of social dynamics, deep changes are expected to affect the community. Immunization, being an emergence as "a continuous, irregular, and unpredictable process of acquisition of non-equivalent (…) properties" gives rise to II type systemic properties.

This passage focuses on the possibility that immunization can eventually allow the community to become steadier through internal changes. What the dynamics previously explored highlight a profile which seems suspended between safety and danger, the conflict between friend and enemy.

Let's turn to our topic: are in/out conflicting poles?

An immune individual cannot be considered an enemy anymore but it is not fully a friend, it is a non-friend. It is a concept that is attested in the Slavic languages, as Vitale underlined (1992) and Schmitt intuitively grasped in *Der Begriff des Politischen.* As the semantic roots from Indo-European domain highlight, an enemy originally refers to someone who stands outside the peaceful community, which is ruled by divine laws. Differently from the enemy, who is permanently in conflict with the State, a non-enemy plays a constructive role for the community because, as Vitale assumes, political friendship can be built only in presence of him (Vitale, 1992: 90). While the enemy questions the existence of the community, the non-friend presents a variety of shades, within a psychological frame that enhances the processes of dialogue/ understanding. As Vitale notes, the "non-friend should be seen as an eminently psychological relation" (1992: 93). Nevertheless, Schmitt had already grasped in his seminal work – as Portinaro argues (1992) – that legacy rooted on a common offspring were too feeble for grounding a valuable theory of political friendship.

I'm now able to formulate my argument and to set my argumentation on more secure ground. At this point in the paper, we should move forward, into the very heart of the immunization process, which will surprisingly reveal a community-like environment more than an exemption place. This premise will bring about a change in the notion of an enemy.

Immunization: a Process of Integration. How the Enemy Builds Up Friend

As Vitale assumes, “the category of friend derives from a psychological process of auto-ascription that is possible only in virtue of the counter opposition” to the enemy (1992: 105, translation is mine). It follows that “it is impossible to elaborate a theory of the political friend (…) that prescinds from the opposition to the enemy.” Thus, a conflict always goes along with the need of sharing a common environment, at least from a psychological perspective. I argue that immunization is very key for highlighting this interconnection. By bringing inside the enemy, immunization clarifies the process that turns hostility into peaceful coexistence, or a permanent transition from conflict to regulation from the systemic outlook. This dynamic maintains a coherent level of organization because of its systemic novelty: it is an emergence, or a II type systemic property, which does not belong to the enemy (out), nor to the community of friends (in) but always need to be fed by both systems. We are at the very heart of the problem investigated in this paper.

It can be expressed by the question: *how does the category of ‘friend’ be built by ‘the enemy inside’?*

The first step is to highlight on *coherence*, which is the process that supports any emergence. In the biological frame of living entities, for instance, health is the state of maximum coherence; on the contrary, any disease gives rise to the isolation of a part, or function, or property of the whole system from the systemic unitary and general coherence. The virus, as a pathogenic agent, by infiltrating within the bodily system as an enemy, disconnects the previous harmonic balance of the bodily system. The loss of coherence clarifies why a process of emergence may be extinguished as the consequence of an inconsistent organization. At the same time, coherence also supports the unitary and integrated response of the system to disturbances/perturbations, avoiding isolation or the independent organization of some parts or functions. Both the innate and the adaptive response of the immune system work as such against the infection.

If the individual 1) is strong enough to react to the virus or 2) a vaccine has been injected into his body, the biological response against the pathogenic agent will not simply destroy it; it will give rise to a reaction that reconnects – in a completely new and different way – functions and properties previously being offended. This leading reaction, within a frame where structural incompleteness is a condition of the process, makes an emergence to be possible. Thus, the enemy, as a process of dissipation and rupture, is expected to provide a stronger coherence in the system.

An enemy could be regarded as a change enabler, an activator of emergence.

We can refer once again to biology, focusing on the parasite/host interaction. The host is commonly perceived as an organism that harbors another living entity inside its specific environment. Worth noting that the Latin word *hostis* resonates in the word *host* with its inner ambiguity of either 1) a guest and 2) a hostile attacker. This set of considerations provides a valuable premise to assume that the process of immunization, where a "friend" of the organism (the host) is targeted by an "enemy" (the pathogen, the virus) is a peculiar battlefield where each attack becomes an integration, in an incessant dynamic that keeps the organism safe or the reverse. From this point of view, immunity cannot be the opposite of a community because integration is a process that lies at the very heart of both. The notion of 'enemy inside' inhabits this environment.

At this point in the discussion, it would be easier to understand why this integration/connection between an *enemy* and a *friend* (of the community) might be highly relevant for understanding how an enemy is expected to lose its destructive potential, turning into a non-friend. As Vitale noted, political friendship can be built through the enemy and only in virtue of this immunization process. If we look at the two poles (enemy/friend) as separate entities that never match or interact, we'll never be able to solve the contradiction. On the contrary, as argued before, they are regarded in terms of open systems that interact. The immune system proves that pathogen/host interactions do not only exist but are part of the process. Criticism can be made, through a question: *how to move from the biology to the classic conflict dynamics?* I'll reply by providing an argument that has been already briefly sketched by philosopher Derrida (1995) and now seems highly valuable to strengthen the idea of the 'enemy inside' as a *trait d'union* between enemy and friend. It recalls, on the political discourse, what has been previously understood in the biological and systemic fields.

In his analysis of Schmitt's *Der Begriff des Politischen*, Derrida assumed that the enemy is an individual who is entirely shaped by the conflict, according to what also Vitale underlined (1992). It is right there in the battlefield, within the crucial space of the frontline, that the foe becomes fully identifiable; however, while the *polemos* builds up the enemy's identity, it also seems to do the reverse, forging a sort of commonality between the two parts in the battlefield. In Derrida's view, this face-to-face condition is expected to delete any difference between enemy and friend. The making of *adversaries* is really what happens in virtue of the polemos, which brings together, as Derrida states "those two are opposed and it provides a historic figure for this polemos that brings enemies together as though they were conjoined in the extreme proximity of face-to-face" (p. 37). In the conflict, in other words, 'enemy' is no more a term that stands in opposition to 'friend'; it turns into an adversary who *participates* in strengthening its identity as well as the one of the other adversaries who are now sharing the conflict experience. On the other hand, this frame highlights on how crucial it is "to construct a distance between soldiers and their enemies" in order "to be able to kill adversaries" (Grossman, 1995).

If we come back to immunization as a conflict that takes place within of the biological system of the individual against the virus, we understand that the enemy (the virus) is defeated when the body assumes some properties of the *enemy* itself, turning into the *adversary* of the virus. Hence, in the immunization battle, the enemy, which is "existentially something different and alien" (Schmitt, 1996: 27) makes its double: the adversary.

CONCLUSION

This paper was intended to focus on the novelty that COVID-19 brought into the discourse about the concept of enemy. As we noticed at the beginning, the metaphors of war are deeply related to the pandemic: what I sought to do, in my investigation, is to turn the limits in understanding the phenomenon into a fruitful resource to understand its opaque ground. I noticed that the concept of the enemy cannot be easily separated from the one of a friend, since the classic Schmitt's theory (1932) to Vitale's investigations on the non-friend, which introduced a more complex understanding of Schmitt traditional divide between (public) enemy, friend and private enemy.

Secondarily, I argued that the very idea of enemy, in the COVID-19 pandemic, should be about the immunization process, that's to say with the battlefield where the conflict against the pathogen coronavirus is performed. Immunity, the condition provided by immunization, is a term that turned from biology into politics and philosophy, in opposition to community. As for the couple enemy/friend, the distinction between these two poles gives rise to a contradiction (Esposito, 1998; 2001). However, if we look at the COVID-19 outbreak scenario, we realize that – at least on the biological ground - immunity is not in conflict with the community. Thus, the idea of an 'enemy inside' which could be a relevant part of the process of immunization, kept on being shaped by the discussion.

A change of paradigm was due, to reach some valuable results. Far from being a universal key for grasping complexity, the systemic perspective might be seen as a toolkit to solve some – not all – traditional philosophical problems, as the enemy/friend dual pole. According to the GST I could argue that immunization, which is a II type systemic property could be regarded as an integration more than an exemption. This idea, gained from the dynamics of dissipative systems can be found also in the biological dynamics of the pathogen/host interactions.

One of the most relevant insights that come from this passage is about the in/out poles, whose interaction is as relevant as their opposition. A further step was to assume that immunization, too, is a process of integration which may be highly relevant to clarify how the enemy builds up the friend, as Schmitt had already shown in his seminal essay (1932) but never developed, and Vitale (1992) integrated with an enlarged perspective on political psychology.

Finally, I noted that conflict is necessary to transform an enemy into an adversary: this is the very basis for making political friendship possible. Pacts can be done between adversaries, because they are a peer in the *polemos*, in virtue of being face-to-face on the frontline. Immunization is not simply the destruction of the foe; it is a more complex process that turns two parts in conflict into adversaries: thus, the enemy does not disappear completely; it turns into an adversary who can be controlled and can enhance the capacity of the reaction of the immune subject. Immunization is the phase in which the enemy is defeated according to a pact with him. Since the virus is an enemy outside the biological body the war cannot be won. What does this phenomenon say to the traditional debate about the concept of the enemy? It highlights the impossibility of making a sharp separation between enemy and friend, as if they were two separated poles, without any communication or any mutual exchange. Through the lens of the General System Thinking, friend and enemy are open systems that interact, especially in the immunization process, a veritable conflict where the two subjects/systems become adversaries. The adversary emerges as a II type systemic property that does not belong to any previous system but cannot be shaped without their mutual interactions.

References

Bilewicz M, Bilewicz A (2012). Who Defines Humanity? Psychological and Cultural Obstacles to Omniculturalism. *Culture & Psychology,* 18(3): 331-344.

Boseley, S. (2020). Coronavirus should be seen as ‘public enemy number one ‘says HO, *The Guardian*. Available at: https://www.theguardian.

com/world/2020/feb/11/coronavirus-vaccine-could-be-ready-in18-months-says-who.

Campi A (ed) (2020). Dopo. Come la pandemia può cambiare la politica, l'economia, la comunicazione e le relazioni internazionali [*How Pandemic Can Change Politics, Economy, and International Relations*], Soveria Mannelli: Rubbettino.

Ceri P, Lorini A (2019). *La costruzione del nemico. Istigazione all'odio in Occidente*. [*The Construction of the Enemy: instilling hate in the West*] Torino: Rosenberg and Sellier.

Derrida J. (1995), *The Gift of Death,* Chicago and London: The University of Chicago Press.

Di Ciaccia F (1985). Sollecitudine e delirio nella peste manzoniana. Studi e ricerche francescane [*Solicitude and Delirium in Manzonian Plague*], 14: 1-245.

Dupré J (2015). Pluralism and Processes in Understanding Human Nature, *Rivista di Filosofia Neoscolastica*, 1-2: 15-28.

Esposito R (1998). *Communitas. Origine e destino della comunità.* [*Communitas: Origin and Destiny of Comminity*]- Torino: Einaudi.

Esposito R (2002). Immunitas. Protezione e negazione della vita. [*Immunitas: Protection and Negation of Life*]- Torino: Einaudi.

Esposito R (2004). *Bios. Biopolitica e filosofia*. [*Bios. Bio-Politica and Philosoph*y] Torino: Einaudi.

Esposito R (2011). *Immunitas.* Cambridge: Poly Press. [*Immunity*.]

Fisogni P (2014). Lone Wolves: Updating the Concept of Enemy in the Social Media Age. *International Journal of Warfare and Terrorism* 4(1): 36-44.

Fisogni P (2014). *Ontologia della speranza*. [*Ontology of Hope*]- Mantova: Gilgamesh.

Fisogni P (2019). The New Front Line (Enhanced). Updating the Concept of Enemy in the Onlife Age. In M Sarfaz (ed.) *Development in Information Security and Cybernetic Wars*. New York: Igi Global: 178-196.

Gell PHG, Coombs RRA (eds.) (1968). *Clinical Aspects of Immunology*. Oxford: Blackwell.

Girard R (1982). *Il capro espiatorio*. [*The Scapegoat*] Milano: Adelphi.

Hunter D (2020). Coronavirus: If We Are in a War Against COVID-19 then we need to know where the enemy is, *The Conversation*, April 2001. Available at: https//theconversation.com/coronavirus-if-we-are-in-a-war-against-covid-19-then-we-need-to-know-where-the-enemy-is-135274.

Gosio N (2020). *Nemici miei. La pervasiva rabbia quotidiana*. [*My Enemies. The Pervasive Daily Rage*] Torino: Einaudi.

Igea, J M (2015). From the Old Immunitas to Modern Immunity: Do We Need a New Name for the Immune System? *Current Immunology Reviews,* 11, 55-65.

Lyon D (2003). *Surveillance After 9/11*. Cambridge: Polity Press.

Lyon D (2007). *Surveillance Studies: An Overview*, Cambridge: Polity Press.

Manzoni A (1984). *Storia della Colonna Infame-Prima redazione, a cura di C. Riccardi*, [*The History of The Infamous Column*] Milano: Mondadori.

Pessa, E. (2013). Emergenza, metastrutture e sistemi gerarchici: verso una nuova teoria generale dei sistemi. In L. Urbani Ulivi (Ed.), *Strutture di mondo. Il pensiero sistemico come specchio di una realtà complessa* (pp. 73-87), [Emergence, Meta-structures, and Hierarchical Systems: Towards a New General System Theory. In: *Structures of World.* Systemic Thinking as a Mirror of a Complex Reality]- Bologna: Il Mulino.

Portinaro P P (1992). Materiali per una storicizzazione della coppia 'amico-nemico,' in G. Miglio (ricerca diretta da), *Amicus (inimicus) Hostis. Le radici concettuali della conflittualità 'privata' e della conflittualità 'politica.'* [*Materials for a Historicization of the 'Friend-Enemy' Couple*] Milano: Giuffrè, 223-306.

Prigogine I (1967). Structure, dissipation, and life. Communication presented at the First International Conference on Theoretical Physics and Biology, Versailles, in *Theoretical Physics and Biology: Proceedings of the First International Conference on Theoretical*

Physics and Biology, Palais des Congrès, Versailles, 26-30 June, 1967 (North-Holland, Amsterdam, 1969).

Prigogine I (1980). *From Being to Becoming: Time and Complexity in the Physical Sciences New York:* W. H. Freeman.

Prigogine I (1999). *Il tempo come principio di sensatezza del cosmo. Intervista a Ilya Prigogine di Vera Fisogni*. A Parte Rei. Available at: http://serbal.pntic.mec.es/~cmunoz11/intervista.pdf [*The Time as a Principle of Sense of the Cosmos. Interview with Ilya Prigogine*]

Schmitt C (2009). Der Begriff des Politischen: Text von 1932 mit einem Vorwort und Drei Corollarien. [*The Concept of the Political: Text from 1932 with a Foreword and Three Corollaries*] Berlin: Dunker & Humblot.

Schmitt C (1996). *The Concept of the Political,* Chicago and London: Chicago University Press.

Vitale A (1992). Il "nemico" nelle lingue slave. Dal concetto di 'nemico' come 'non-amico' alla conflittualità 'privata' e 'politica,' in G. Miglio (ricerca diretta da), *Amicus (inimicus) Hostis*. Le radici concettuali della conflittualità 'privata' e della conflittualità 'politica.' Milano: Giuffrè, 87-216 [The "Enemy" in Slavic Languages. From the Concept of 'Enemy' as 'Non-friend' to 'Private' and 'Political' Conflict. In: *Amicus (inimicus) Hostis*. The Conceptual Roots of 'Private' Conflict and 'Political' Conflict.]

Urbani Ulivi, L. (2015). (Ed.). Strutture di mondo. Il pensiero sistemico come specchio di una realtà complessa, Bologna: Il Mulino. [*Structures of World. Systemic Thinking as a Mirror of a Complex Reality*]

Urbani Ulivi, L. (2013). *La struttura dell'umano. Linee di un'antropologia sistemica*, In L. [*The structure of the human. Lines of a systemic anthropology*]

Urbani Ulivi (Ed.), *Strutture di mondo* (pp. 231-247), Bologna: Il Mulino. [*World structures*]

Urbani Ulivi, L. (2019). Mind and Body. Whose? Philosophy of Mind and the Systemic Approach. In L. Urbani Ulivi (Ed.). *The Systemic Turn in*

Human and Natural Sciences. A Rock in The Pond (pp. 185-205), Cham, Switzerland: Springer.

Urbani Ulivi L. (2019). *First Steps towards a Systemic Ontology. Systemics of Incompleteness and Quasi-Systems*. In Minati G, Abram MR, Pessa E, editors.

Vitiello G (2019). The World Opacity and Knowledge. In L. Urbani Ulivi (Ed.), *The Systemic Turn in Human and Natural Sciences. A Rock in The Pond* (pp. 41-51). Cham, Switzerland: Springer.

In: Emotionality of COVID-19 ISBN: 978-1-53619-534-7
Editors: M. Korstanje and S. Adrian © 2021 Nova Science Publishers, Inc.

Chapter 4

PANDEMIC, INTERNET AND EMOTIONS: POLITICS OF SENSIBILITIES AND COMMODIFICATION OF AUDIENCES

Pedro Lisdero[1,*] and Marion Fonrouge[2,†]
[1]CIECS - CONICET and UNC//UNVM//CIES
[2]University of Palermo, Buenos Aires, Argentina

ABSTRACT

On March 11, 2019, the World Health Organization declared the status of a pandemic for the rapid expansion of COVID-19. In a short period of time, the daily lives of billions of people around the world would never be the same: the successive strategies that were adopted in different countries implied significant changes in most of the subjects' daily experiences, from the way of working to the family relationship itself. Most of the situations of interactions in the context of the pandemic are carried out in virtual contexts, and specifically through social networks. Thus, COVID-19 is imposed as a recurring "topic of discussion": WhatsApp groups, Facebook, etc. are filled with messages

* Corresponding Author's E-mail: pedrolisdero@gmail.com.
† Corresponding Author's E-mail: mfacultad5@gmail.com.

and discussions about it. Thinking in terms of social research, it is possible to imagine a Big Data strategy to analyze the traceability of messages, and to map the density of the circulation of information. However, it is also possible to ask ourselves some questions that seek the qualitative meanings of the practice of receiving and re-sending messages related to the subject, while taking into account its relationship with their form. In this direction, the objective of this chapter is to analyze the emotions linked to the interactions in social networks associated with COVID-19. To do this, we applied a self-administered survey to 307 respondents in 17 European countries, selected using the snowball sampling technique between March 17th and April 18th, where we inquired about how people feel when they receive/send information related to the pandemic. Given the multiple possible interpretations, we are interested in linking some discussions around digital labor, that is, the ability of social networks to market to an audience. This means emphasizing one of the ways these media have, in the framework of the renewed and massive situations of digital interaction, of capturing people's energies and transforming them into merchandise (Fuchs, 2014). The analysis focuses on the fact that what is commercialized is the willingness to be part of a group that receives messages, so it is not enough to just know the quantifiable dimension of the action of forwarding, but also what is at stake is the relationship between the objective field and the willingness of the subjects to be part of these audiences. Therefore, beyond the re-production of the practice (whether it is re-sent or not re-sent), we are interested here in exploring how the qualitative sense that agents give to it could be associated with policies of digital sensibilities (Scribano and Lisdero, 2019). That is, perceptions framed in specific regimes of sensibilities that allow connecting bodily geometries with grammars of action (Scribano, 2017) that have a specific support and content in the digital field. This allows us to advance in the description of "platform sensibilities" as a sign of the ongoing social structuration processes.

1. Introduction

On March 11th, 2019, the World Health Organization declared the status of a pandemic for the rapid expansion of COVID-19. In a short period of time, the daily lives of billions of people around the world would never be the same: the successive strategies that were adopted in different countries implied significant changes in most of the subjects' daily experiences, from the way of working to the family relationship itself.

Most of the situations of interactions in the context of the pandemic are carried out in virtual contexts, and specifically through social networks. Thus, COVID-19 is imposed as a recurring "topic of discussion": WhatsApp groups, Facebook, etc. they filled with messages and discussions about it. Thinking in terms of social research, it is possible to imagine a Big Data strategy to analyze the traceability of messages, and to map the density of the circulation of information. However, it is also possible to ask ourselves some questions that seek the qualitative meanings of the practice of receiving and re-sending messages related to the subject, while taking into account its relationship with their form. In this direction, the objective of this chapter is to analyze the emotions linked to the interactions in social networks associated with COVID-19. To do this, we applied a self-administered survey to 307 respondents in 17 European countries, selected using the snowball sampling technique between March 17th and April 18th, where we asked about how people feel when they receive/send information related to the pandemic. Given the multiple possible interpretations, we are interested in linking some discussions around digital labor, that is, the ability of social networks to commodify an audience (Fuchs, 2014). This means emphasizing one of the ways these media have, in the framework of the renewed and massive situations of digital interaction, of capturing people's energies and transforming them into a commodity. The analysis focuses on the fact that what is commercialized is the willingness to be part of a group that receives messages, so it is not enough to just know the quantifiable dimension of the action of forwarding, but also what is at stake is the relationship between the objective field and the willingness of the subjects to be part of these audiences. Therefore, beyond the re-production of the practice (whether it is re-sent or not re-sent), we are interested here in exploring how the qualitative sense that agents give to it could be associated with policies of digital sensibilities (Scribano and Lisdero, 2019). That is, perceptions framed in specific regimes of sensibilities that allow connecting bodily geometries with grammars of action (Scribano, 2017) that have a specific support and content in the digital field. This allows us to advance in the description of “platform sensibilities” as a sign of the ongoing social structuration processes.

2. The Emotional Commodification of the Audience

Given the breadth of the problem linked to the relationship between emotions and pandemic, we have focused on the specificity of digital labor, and its links with the processes of commodification enabled in digital media. To do so, we will rely on the analysis of empirical data built from the "Covid and Emotions" Survey (CIES). This study was undertaken using a non-probabilistic, exploratory design, where the snowball technique was used for the construction of the sample. A self-administered form was applied, elaborated from the "google form" tool, which contains a series of closed and open questions related to the relationship between emotions and COVID-19 (in addition to other general information). Thus, a total of 307 responses were collected between March 17th and April 18th. Most of the responses are concentrated in Italy (152 cases, or 49.5%), Spain (62 cases, or 20.2%), France (33 cases, or 10.6%), United Kingdom (11 cases, 3.5%), Portugal (11 cases, 3.5%), and Russia (10 cases, 3.2%). Other countries from which responses were received are Belgium, Austria, Germany, Greece, Ireland, Sweden, Hungary, Finland, Luxembourg, Czech Republic and the Netherlands. The age of the respondents ranges from 17 to 73 years, grouped as follows: 23.1% are between 17 and 25 years; 32.2% are between 26 and 35 years; 24.8% are between 36 and 45 years; 13% are between 46 and 55 years; 4.2% are between 56 and 65 years, and 2.6% are 66 years of age or older (about 57% of the sample is between 26 and 46 years). Sixty-four percent (64%) of the respondents are women, while 33.2% are men (1.9% responded "Prefer not to say"). With respect to educational level, 89% of the sample has completed university studies. The main occupations recorded are: "Professional, technical and related worker" (28.3%), "Student" (27.7%), "Government/public sector" (14%), "Administrative, managerial" (9.4%), "Unemployed/looking for work" (4.6%), "Other service worker" (3.6%), "Sales" (3.3%), "Home-based worker/subcontractor" (2.6%), and "Housework" (1.6%).

In this chapter we will focus on two questions: "Have you re-sent information related to COVID-19 through WhatsApp, We-Chat, Facebook, Twitter, Instagram or other social networks ?"; and "Why?." Next, we advance making explicit an analytical proposal, and presenting some preliminary results that make it possible to draw some interpretative lines regarding the proposed objectives.

2.1. Digital Labor, Audience Commodification, and Emotional Work: Contributions from Sociology of Sensibilities

Many of the interaction situations in the context of the pandemic are carried out through digital media, and specifically through social networks. Within this framework, COVID-19, as well as all the "news" that were installed about it, was imposed as a "topic of discussion": WhatsApp groups, Facebook, Twitter, Instagram, TikTok, and in general the most popular social networks were invaded by messages and discussions about it.

A first interesting question could be "what does these media, which we summarize here as Social Networks (WhatsApp, Facebook, Twitter, etc.) have in common?" In what sense does the capacity of digital media to "commodify an audience" expand from the practices involved in the use of these social networks? Recovering the analysis of Dallas Smythes (1977) on the notion of audience commodity, Fuchs (2014) observes:

> "(…) the rise of user-generated content, free access social networking platforms and other free access platforms that yield profit by online advertisement—a development subsumed under categories such as Web 2.0, social software and social networking sites—the web seems to come close to accumulation strategies employed by capital on traditional

mass media like TV or radio. Users who upload photos and other images, write wall postings and comments, send mail to their contacts, accumulate friends or browse other profiles on Facebook constitute an audience commodity that is sold to advertisers. The difference between the audience commodity on traditional mass media and on the Internet is that in the latter case the users are also content producers, there is user-generated content and the users engage in permanent creative activity, communication, community building and content production. That the users are more active on the Internet than in the reception of TV or radio content is due to the decentralized structure of the Internet that allows many-to-many communication. Because of the permanent activity of the recipients and their status as prosumers, we can say that in the case of corporate social media the audience commodity is an Internet prosumer commodity. (Fuchs 2010b)" (100)

Within the framework of a sociology of sensibilities[1], the discussion raised at the crossroads between digital labor[2] and the commodification of

[1] Schematically, we could say that the aforementioned Sociology of Sensibilities is inscribed in a particular perspective (Scribano, 2017; Scribano and Lisdero, 2019) that recovers the centrality of the body/emotions in social theory in order to understand the current processes of social structuration. The idea of body seeks to stress an individual body (bio-physical substrate), a subjective body and a social body. Emotions can be seen as the puzzle that comes as an action and effect of feeling or sensation: these situate in the states of feeling the world that allow the organization of perceptions associated with socially constructed forms of sensations. From this we understand "bodily energy" as the result of the exchange of physiological systems and biological processes associated with the durability of the individual body, but also as the (insubstantial) substratum of the processes of value creation in societies. The work in Western capitalist history can be historicized in an important dimension of its expression, starting from the constant re-inventions of the corporal energies, in consonance with the metabolic mechanisms linked to the accumulation regimes. Within this framework of general understanding, we think that the consequences and central effects of the relationships between Society 4.0, digital labor and the social structuration process are the changes in the politics of sensibilities, understood as the set of cognitive-affective social practices tending to the production, management and reproduction of horizons of action, disposition and cognition. (Scribano, 2017, Scribano and Lisdero, 2019).

[2] Three analytical nodes are differentiated in the available research on the notion of digital labour: (a) the discussion about the objects of expropriation in digital processes, highlighting the differential place occupied by the body and knowledge within the framework of a renewed discussion about the theory of value (Fuchs 2014; Fumagalli, 2015; Dyer-Witheford 2015; Morini and Fumagalli 2010; Huws 2016; Andrejevic 2012; Fisher 2012; Fisher and Fuchs 2015; Heam 2010; Vercellone 2006); (b) discussions about work processes and their material supports (time/space coordination of productive interactions), in the framework of which the notions of "Prosumption" (Ritzer and Jurgenson 2010), or "Playbour/Gamebour" (Arwid 2015), "free labour" (Newfoundland

audiences opens up the possibility of asking ourselves about the bodily energies that support these renewed processes of capitalist accumulation. For this we need to incorporate the notion of emotional work: early on, A. Hoschchild (1983) analyzed flight attendants and insurance salesmen by taking as a focus of reflection the connections between the emotions produced in work and the processes of value production. The author proposes that there is an institutionalization of the emotional order of the work environment on the intimate sphere, where the management of affects in the labor world begins to possess a certain predetermined and coercive character. Emotions are no longer elaborated from a discreet and personal management, and become instead a work that is marketed to the public. Precisely his study shows that many workers now do not simply sell their physical strength, nor their knowledge or rational capacity, but they also place their emotions on the market. Taking up Hoschild's idea, we are interested here in asking about the expansion and mutation of this trend, specifically in the context of the expansion of digital labor.

It would be impossible in this space to expand on the various responses that have been offered regarding this relationship (digital labor - emotional work): we ourselves have provided some analytical keys in order to make explicit the possible contributions of a sociology of sensibilities in the complexities of the notion of digital labor (Scribano and Lisdero, 2019). In this direction, the centrality of emotional work in our societies could be connected to the observations that Fuchs makes about the processes of value creation in digital labor assumed in social networks. In this regard, Fuchs notes:

2013; Kosnik 2013) "unpaid labour" (Fuchs, 2014), and cooperative/collaborative work (Meil and Kirov, 2017) are discussed. The idea of a "platform capitalism" (Cingolani, 2016) characterized by the growing place of the so-called "sharing economy" (Irani 2015; Cingolani 2016) emerges here. (c) Finally, a third group of researches deals with the constitution of the subjects that work, highlighting intensification, dependence (global), feminization and neo-taylorization (Huws, 2016), precariousness (Dyer-Witheford, 2015) and heterogeneity (types of organization, environments, contractual relations) (Fuchs and Sandoval, 2015). The perspective proposed here starting from the discussion about the body/emotions linked to digital labour, and seeks to establish the mediations between the vitality of bodies and emotions as an object of exploitation.

> "Whereas wage labour is coerced by the threat of physical violence (the threat is death because of the lack of being able to purchase and consume goods), audience labour is coerced by ideological violence (the threat is to have fewer social contacts because of missing information from the media and missing communication capacities that are needed for sustaining social relations). (…) If for example people stop using Facebook and social networking sites, they may miss certain social contact opportunities. They can refuse to become a Facebook worker, just like an employee can refuse to work for a wage, but they may as a consequence suffer social disadvantages in society. Commercial media coerce individuals to use them." (2014: 90-91)
>
> "(…) Marx argues that for being considered a productive worker, "it is no longer necessary for the individual himself to put his hand to the object; it is sufficient for him to be an organ of the collective labourer, and to perform any one of its subordinate functions" (ibid., 643–644). This means that productive labour understood this way implies that a worker who contributes to a "social product" that is controlled by a capitalist and is the "joint product of a collective labourer" (ibid., 643) is an exploited worker, no matter if s/he receives a wage for it or not. S/he is part of a collective or social worker. (…) "(2014: 109)
>
> "Social media users are double objects of commodification: they are commodities themselves and through this commodification their consciousness becomes, while online, permanently exposed to commodity logic in the form of advertisements. Most online time is advertising time "(2014: 101)

In the quoted fragments, we highlight three elements: 1. the extortion associated with the "ideological violence" to which the "digital workers" are subjected is experienced from the "fewer social contacts" and "the suffering social disadvantages," which puts the "body" at the center of the scene as the origin of social relations, and as the privileged "platform" where the social processes of production begin and end; 2. the productivity of connection, as well as the exploitation associated with the mutations of the value chain, needs to be explained from a collective body - a "living organ" that as the engine of life is captured in its productivity from a sociability that requires a particular "way of being"; and 3. precisely this is what we could read behind the idea of "commodification of consciousness," a subsidiary of the digital moment of the "consciousness Industry" (Hans Magnus Enzensberger, in Fuchs 2014). Accommodating the collective body of digital workers to the demands of the 4.0 “consciousness industry” implies a self-production that we could associate with “emotional work.” The key to this association is to think about embodied consciousnesses: emotions connect the sensitive and biographical expression of bodies with the social trends from which these bodies are marked. Contrary to the notions that consecrate the body-mind division, our proposal lies in connecting digital labor with emotional work to emphasize that affects are re-invented as "productive muscle." This has a differential characteristic in a world where social networks have colonized the internal planet: this "emotional muscle" cannot be thought of without the digital context. Thus, thinking about emotions in the context of social networks allows us to take a relational look at the “collective body” of digital workers as the (insubstantial) substratum of the processes of value creation and valorization from the affects that are commodified in/by social networks. We propose here to think about the commodification of affects as a necessary element to understand the "commodification of audience."

In order to operationalize this discussion, and advance in an analytical approach that allows us to put it in the context of some emerging empirical evidence, we will recover the two questions referred to in the survey on "Emotions and Covid-19." In this direction, we could think that the first question (Have you re-sent information related to "COVID-19" on social networks?) is an indicator of the processes of "commodification of audiences" in a double sense: in the first place it is an objective indicator of the potential of future communications, as a multiplier possibility to demarcate and build the audience (by amplifying interactions). Secondly, even when the subjects do not re-send the message, they are still not exempt from reproducing audience commodification, as long as they remain interacting in the digital medium, and therefore, building (possibly) data that are captured, processed and sold as commodities by the corporations that control the digital interactions. We will call this second dimension "limited re-production" of the audience, to differentiate it from the alluded to "extended re-production," although we must also clarify that the range of possibilities of digital relations should also include the possibility that the subjects can remove this logic from the commodity. However, we will not analyze this dimension here, since our objective is to explore the "emotional environment" that can be linked to the commodification of the audience.

It is not enough just to know whether or not the subjects re-sent messages: one may not have re-sent but even receiving it is part of a chain whose objective conditions of reproduction far exceed the calculation of individual behaviors. In other words, what is at stake is the relationship between the objective field and the willingness of the subjects to be part of those audiences. Therefore, beyond the re-production of the practice (whether or not to re-send), exploring the meaning that the agents imprint on it is more interesting from our perspective, inasmuch as in this set of dispositions they express the objective conditions of this chain of value production.

Thus, the information contained in the second question is important: "why did you decide to send/not send?." Since this is an open question, we chose to recategorize the answers received by registering them as an indicator of the "policies of sensibilities," that is, by differentiating in them (only for analytical purposes) the cognitive content from the affective one. The first dimension grouped the responses according to four emerging logics: 1. "Logic of Communication" - the meaning of the action is related to different motives aimed at facilitating communication, clarifying information, denouncing fakes news, avoiding "noise" in communication, and so on e.g., "to inform people about fake news"; 2. "Logic of knowledge" - the sense of action is related to the search for intervention in the processes from which to approach the "truth" (about what is happening) e.g., "share knowledge"; 3. "Logic of responsibility" - the sense of action emphasizes the consequences of individual actions aimed at the achievement of the "common good" e.g., "because I don't want to help spread fear"; and 4. "Logic of imitation" - the reason for action is to ensure a minimum degree of interaction without reflecting on the meaning of the action, imitation, or entertainment e.g., "to have a conversation."

The second dimension mentioned (affective) was reconstructed by identifying six groups of "feelings practices": 1. "Knowledge/awareness" - this includes feelings practices associated with the need to "become aware" (e.g., "because it's important for people who don't know what the problems are"); 2. "Trust" - sensations linked to trust/distrust with respect to people, institutions, etc. (e.g., "I'm not sure of its truth"); 3. Feeling useful/Care/Interest/Solidarity-Hope" - a set of feeling practices that, although they have certain peculiarities, all highlight the personal affective involvement in the consideration and possibility of action oriented towards an "other" (e.g., "I feel like adding some help for the society"); 4. "Love/friendship" - sensations where what is emphasized is the bond of love or friendship (e.g., "to inform my friend about some topic"); 5. "Fear/Anxiety" (e.g., "I'm against panic"); 6. "Entertainment": practices of feeling associated with the sensation of entertainment (e.g., "For sharing ... coronavirus jokes").

We would like to offer some clarifications here: the construction of categories for the dimensions mentioned was undertaken aiming at the greatest capacity for grouping them, fulfilling each one of the options the necessary characteristics of exhaustiveness and mutual exclusion. In this sense, the imputation of meaning in the re-coding process emphasized the identification of the cognitive logics and "feeling practices" predominant in the expressions made by the subjects in the form. The proposed categories constitute an analytical effort to reduce the complexity of meaning that these expressions embody.

Finally, before presenting some preliminary results from the analytical proposal presented, it would be relevant to say something more about our point of arrival, an issue that we could discuss based on the relationship between policies of sensibilities – the geometry of bodies and grammars of digital actions[3]. In other words, we would like to ask ourselves here in

---

[3] The notion of the geometry of bodies refers us to the dispositions that "shape" society from particular coordinates of the social positioning of bodies. For its part, the idea of the

what sense the constructed information informs us about the perceptions that the subjects have about their practice (condensing and paradigmatic linked to networks and coronaviruses), and how those perceptions are framed in specific regimes of sensibilities that allow connecting geometries with possible digital grammars.

As a summary, the analytical proposal presented here could be summarized as follows (Figure 1):

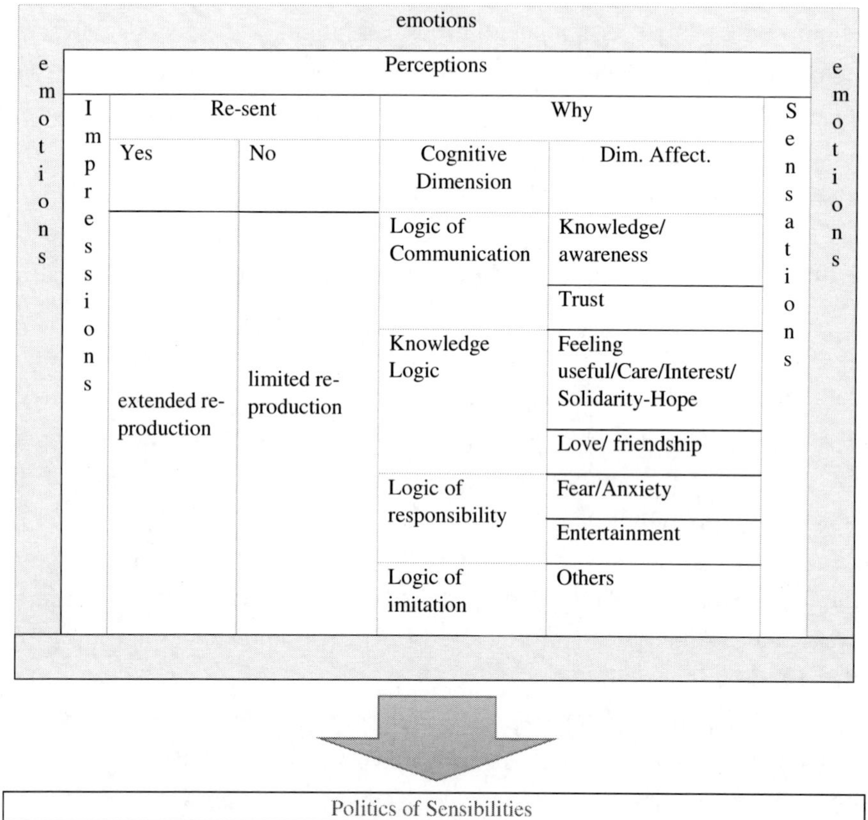

Figure 1. Analytical proposal.

"grammar of actions" allows us to access the common ways of giving meaning to social practices in-and by-the bodies referred to (Scribano, 2004b).

2.2. Presentation of Data and Preliminary Readings

The study shows that a significant majority of people (71% of the respondents) resent messages linked to "COVID-19" through their social networks (Figure 2). If we take the reasons for these actions as a group between those who forwarded and those who did not forward, we find that:

- Regarding the "Cognitive Dimension" (Figure 3) of the practice, the "Logic of Communication" stands out, gathering 51.5% of the cases (158 answers), followed by the "Logic of Responsibility," with 20.2% of the cases (62 answers), while the "Logic of Knowledge" and "Logic of Imitation" account for 13.4% (41 answers) and 8.8% (27 answers) of the cases.
- The "Affective Dimension" (Figure 4) shows that most of the responses concentrated on the sensations of "Knowledge/Awareness" (31.6%, 97 answers), "Trust" (20.2%, 62 answers), "Love/Friendship" (16%, 49 answers) and "Feel useful/Caring/Interest/Solidarity-hope" (12.4%, 38 answers). All these emotions grouped together concentrate then more than 80% of the answers. Finally, less frequently the respondents mention "Fear/Anxiety" (6.8%, 21 answers) and "Entertainment" (5.5%, 17 answers).

An interesting appreciation arises from the comparison of responses between those who re-send and those who do not. If we look at the cognitive content (Figure 5) of the practice associated with re-sending, we find that most of the responses are distributed uniformly across all categories, from which we could say that the "cognitive dimension" is not a significant factor in this action. This is not the case with what we call here the "Logic of Imitation," where we assume that a smaller set in the sample (13.4% of the total), which brings together motives linked to "keeping in touch," or deliberately seeking to "have some conversation" or "entertain/be entertained," predominantly brings into play this "cognitive dimension" of the action when re-sending messages.

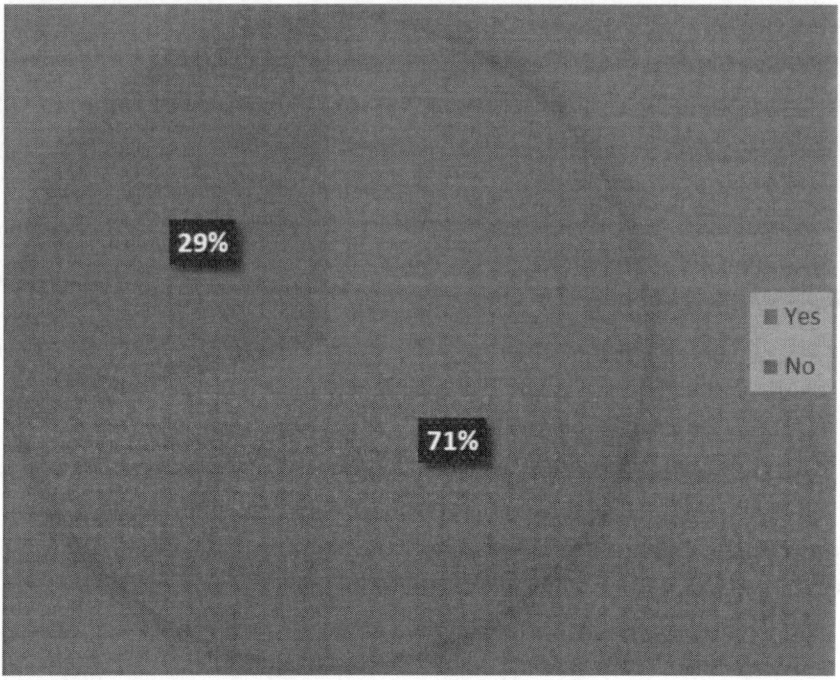

Source: Own elaboration. Survey "Emotions and COVID" (CIES).

Figure 2. Have you re-sent information related to "COVID-19" through Social Networks?

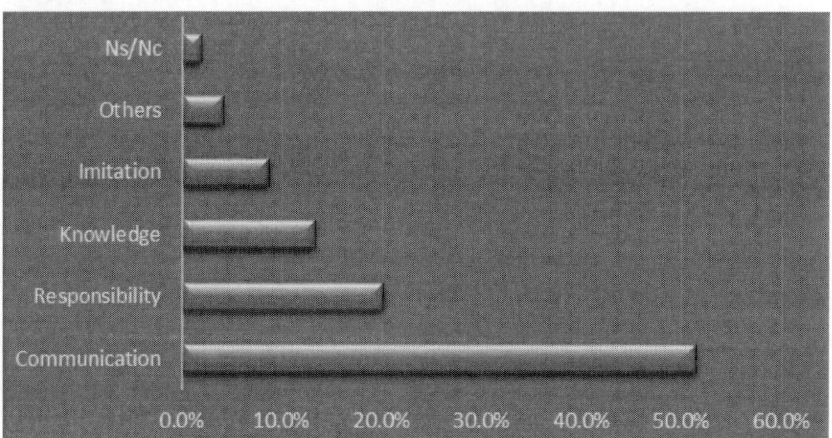

Source: Own elaboration. Survey "Emotions and COVID" (CIES).

Figure 3. Cognitive dimensión.

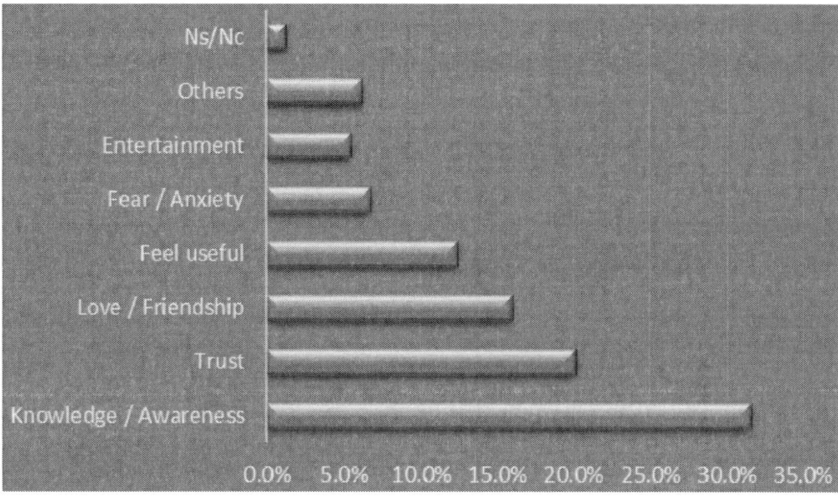

Source: Own elaboration. Survey "Emotions and COVID" (CIES).

Figure 4. Affective dimension.

If we pay attention to the affective content (Figure 6) of the practice, we find that the re-sending variable constitutes a factor that brings together two well-differentiated groups of "feeling practices": the action of re-sending is significantly associated with "Knowledge/Awareness," "Feel useful/Caring/Interest/Solidarity-hope," "Love/Friendship," and "Entertainment"; while "non-re-sending" seems to be associated with "Trust" and "Fear/Anxiety."

	Communication	Knowledge	Responsibility	Imitation / Entertainment	Others	Ns/Nc	
Yes	53.7%	12.4%	19.7%	11.5%	1.4%	1.4%	100%
No	46.1%	15.7%	21.3%	2.2%	11.2%	3.4%	100%

Source: Own elaboration. Survey "Emotions and COVID" (CIES).

Figure 5. Re-sent/ Cognitive Dimension.

	Knowledge / Awareness	Trust	Feel useful	Love / Friendship	Fear / Anxiety	Entertainment	Other	Ns/Nc	
Yes	38.5%	12.4%	15.1%	22.0%	1.8%	7.3%	2.3%	0.5%	100%
No	14.6%	39.3%	5.6%	1.1%	19.1%	1.1%	15.7%	3.4%	100%

Source: Own elaboration. Survey "Emotions and COVID" (CIES).

Figure 6. Re-sent/Affective Dimension.

It is important to emphasize at this point that the "affective dimension" seems to have a certain preeminence in explaining the action of forwarding/non-forwarding. If we observe the links between the cognitive and affective dimensions (Figure 7 and Figure 8) we can see some associations that qualify the alluded preeminence:

- The category that brings together a series of practices of feeling associated with fun and entertainment are linked, from the action of forwarding, with the "Logic of Imitation." That is to say, there is here a two-way connection between the cognitive and affective dimensions that is condensed in the action of re-sending. This speaks to us of the power, embodied in the expanded reproduction of audiences as the balance of the action, of the vertigo produced by the extortion of staying outside the digital-emotional world as a univocal feature of the politics of sensibilities.
- The practices of feeling linked to "awareness" and "love/friendship" seem to be the most frequent among those who forwarded messages as a way of intervening in the communicational process. On the other hand, feeling useful, supportive, hopeful, etc., explains a great part of the sensations of those who re-sent messages looking for some sense linked to the "common good." Both groups of sensations, as a whole, inform us about the horizon of the action embodied in the subjects, which is structured as the emotional basis of "the possible" in this digital world. In the face of the ominous nature of communicational processes, the need to become aware of and "care for" those close to us, to initiate solidarity actions, etc., emerges as sensations that

paradoxically are articulated with the deliberate intention of intervening in communicational processes by amplifying them, or looking for the "common good" by reproducing the practices of differential appropriation of information (not only as a common good but also as a strategic one).

- Finally, the feeling of trust (or lack of trust) describes the emotional state of those who decided not to forward messages, orienting the effects of their practices both in the communicational logic, and in the processes from which it approaches the "truth" ("Logic of Knowledge"). Fear and anxiety characterize the sentimental practices of those who did not send messages, looking to influence both the communicative process and participate in the construction of the "common good." In general, this group of sensations seems to structure two opposite poles (on the one hand confidence and on the other fear/anxiety) that give us insights about uncertainty as a central component of emotionality. This emotionality could be associated with "paralysis," "immobility" as a balance of personal experiences. Not to forward, "not to do" is not synonymous with destitution of the value chain of the audience as a commodity, in such a way that those who pretend "a certain quietness" as a way of "resistance to the "communicational logic," or those who due to fear or anxiety did not dare to forward the messages, are also a "transmission pulley" of the limited re-production of the audiences.

Gathering the tendencies that are described, we can advance in some statements of sense anticipation that allow us to understand how this particular association of cognitive and affective elements can be read as a particular configuration of the politics of sensibilities that underlies the digital practice. These policies constitute an interesting reading key regarding the predispositions with which subjects intervene in the interactions mediated by social networks.

	Entertainment		Love /Friendship		Feel useful		Knowledge/ Awareness		Trust		Fear/ Anxiety	
	Y	**N**	**Y**	**N**	**Y**	**N**	**Y**	**N**	**Y**	**N**	**Y**	**N**
Imitation	16	1	7				2	10				1
Communication			29			9	55	3		42		8
Knowledge				1	3		11		6	11	1	
Responsibility			5	6	22	3	16			3		11
Total	17		48		37		97		62		21	
	Re-sent								Not- re-sent			

Source: Own elaboration. Survey "Emotions and COVID" (CIES).

Figure 7. Re-sent/Affective Dimension/Cognitive Dimension.

Reproduction Amplified		Re-production limited	
Knowledge/Awareness	Communication		
Love/Friendship	Communication	Trust	Communication/Knowledge
Feel Useful	Responsibility	Fear/Anxiety	Responsibility
Entertainment	Imitation		

Source: Own elaboration. Survey "Emotions and COVID" (CIES).

Figure 8. Politics of Sensibilities.

The first consideration arises from the question of what is the bodily disposition to participate in these kinds of digital interactions? How do these interactions occur? The data presented lead us to think that, beyond rational calculation, and framed in a series of specific cognitive logics, the digital practice in/by social networks involves a way of being for others. In other words, "being" in the expanding digital world increasingly implies "being" in social networks, and this presupposes, in addition to many other "skills," being able to "get emotional." Thus, a first point to note is that the affective dimension of the practice which refers to the interplay between the individual's sensations and social emotions seems to invade the cognitive contents with different senses, constituting a kind of "compass" that allows the individual to "navigate" the digital world.

Thus, the "logic of communication," as the predominant cognitive component (both in forwarding actions and in non-forwarding actions) appears to be traversed by various practices of feeling that underlie the communicational field. We can think in this respect that by sharing information an affective content is generated with multiple senses, all of which contribute to elaborate the "viral" dimension of the pandemic as an effect of "ideological violence" (Fuchs, 2014). That is to say, the pandemic constitutes (among other dimensions) first of all an "emotional product" that threatens and extorts those who cannot live it affectively in the networks. The irreversible balance of this practice is a world where the production, circulation and consumption of information-emotion turned into commodity is expanded and consecrated.

This refers directly to the notion of "audience commodification," but from the observation of a specific feature that emphasizes the place occupied by emotions: the data presented announce that the practices of feeling seem to organize the perceptions linked to the cognitive associated with them, constituting in themselves a condition and at the same time a specific content of the relationships in/by social networks. The substratum of value takes the form of the body's affective expression as a reservoir of motives for being in the network. Thus, the idea of production, circulation and "consumption" of information opens the way not only to the image of the "prosumer," but centrally to an "emotional prosumer." The notion of an "affective community" (Ahmed, 2019), as a concept that analyzes the function that emotions have in the construction of collective practices, leads us to think that digital affective exchanges build an "emotional platform" that works by organizing the metabolized energy flows in the processes of audience commodification.

The commoditization of emotions (as a process of delimitation and management of the practices of feeling) associated with the commoditization of audiences, provides the quality of "ambivalence" as a characteristic feature that ensures the effectiveness of these processes in digital contexts. As we observe, there is no difference in the cognitive logics that explain the passage from forwarding to not forwarding: however, the prevalence of certain sensations over the same logics builds a "plus" that allows agents to place themselves in the social world, and the process of audience commodification to expand with different values. Ahmed (2019) suggests that emotions are public, since they are constructed and signified through a collective imaginary. Based on this idea, she makes an analogy with Marx's vision of the movement of money and material goods, to develop the concept of "affective economies," which refers to the way emotions "circulate" and are distributed both in the psyche and in society. Re-appropriating this idea, and putting it in relation to what has been discussed about the commodification of audiences as well as the possibility of thinking from a sociology of sensibilities, social emotions appear as that "plus" associated with sensations, which draw the conditions of operation of the "digital affective communities."

In this direction, the cognitive dimension of the practice informs us about a specific content of the regime of sensibilities as a condition of possibility of these "communities." A transversal look at the cognitive logics presented allows us to observe that what we here call "logic of communication," "of responsibility," and "of knowledge" are configured in the answers of the agents as a way of finding understanding about certainties, and the ways in which these are constructed and distributed. The fact that this cognitive framework is completed with the "logic of imitation" helps us to think that what is at stake is a profound process of reconfiguration of sociabilities, since this whole set of senses puts the "connection," already stripped of its technological garb, at the center of the scene as a condition of the collective body.

However, as we have been observing, if part of the expressed experiences refer us to a mutation of the sociabilities, another part of them refers us to the sensibilities as a central component for understanding this metamorphosis. In this direction, the preeminence of the affective dimension does not respond to an ontological consideration, but rather to an analytical one. It seems to be these explored sensations that orient the "connection" in a double sense: as a way of meaning for the cognitive dimension of the practice, as well as a "plus" that allows an interpretation of the content that constitutes the social emotions as a central component of the regime of sensitivities in course.

CONCLUSION

As an opening we would like to take up again the idea of "platform sensibilities" (Scribano and Lisdero, 2019) to refer to the cognitive-affective state linked - at least - to the following characteristics. In the first place, we should think of this particular state of the "politics of sensibilities" as processes extended in the "here and now" of labor times/spaces, but which operate in an expansive way from the mediations that enable relationships in/through the internet. Thus, as a regime, it stands out for the "intimacy" of the mechanisms that work as a necessary gear for the fluid deployment of the "digital production chain" ("audience commodification").

In this sense, sensibilities of platform imply a particular body policy, where sensitive terminals are processed by the phenomenal capacity of digital sensors to capture the creative forces of the bodies. This requires us to think beyond the processes of "consciousness" centered in the "brain," opening up questions about the complexity of the vital energies that are re-invented in a social body as a surface for the exploitation of digital processes. At the same time, these sensibilities also imply a "politics of emotions" that, as an accepted form of "feeling" oneself with respect to a range of expected practices, is related to a particular potential capacity to act on "others." These social emotions, connected to the sensations experienced by the agents (as we develop), constitute the conditions of digital labor. That is, they come as the mechanisms that occlude the corporal trace of digital energies from the affective tension that orient the perceptions in a "beyond" of the digital processes.

In this work, then, we have tried to move away from dichotomous models in the understanding of emotions, organizing the data from certain continuities of the process of commodification, and following a certain analogy in the tensions between technology and the body. We resynchronize the notion of the body in the context of digital interactions from the basic certainty that if the "instruments" we use change, so do bodily sensations. The individual "supports" (in the Weberian sense) new forms of relationship, becoming the embodiment of digital technology. There are different ways of taking over the world, and technology is a new "logic of proximity." The body becomes an instrument, and in a way, it is a technology of communication with the other: the acts of bodily speech are modified according to the instruments, rewriting the body as the territory of life (and therefore of the productive processes in which it is inscribed). The problem of capitalism in societies 4.0 (Scribano and Lisdero, 2019) is the colonization of human and non-human nature, and "the digital" is no different from life. However, in the amplification of its re-productive processes, the logic of the commodity in-corporates the expressive forms of "being" in the digital world as a privileged component: being productive today is not only about "adapting" to the use of digital technologies, but above all about being willing to get emotional (not in any way).

REFERENCES

Ahmed, S. (2019) *La promesa de felicidad. Una crítica cultural al imperativo de la alegría.* [*The promise of happiness: a cultural critique to the mandate of happiness*]. Buenos Aires: Caja Negra Editora.

Arwid, L. (2015) A Contribution to a Critique of the Concept Playbour. In E. Fisher & C. Fuchs (Eds.), *Reconsidering Value and Labour in the Digital Age* (pp. 63–79). Westminster: Palgrave Macmillan.

Cingolani, P. (2016). *Capitalismo de plataforma: nuevas tecnologías de la comunicación e internacionalización del trabajo.* [*Platform capitalism: new communication technologies and the internationalisation of labour*]. Boletín Onteaiken, 22, 42–47.

Dyer-Witheford, N. (2015) *Cyber-proletariat. Global Labour in the Digital Vortex.* London: Pluto Press.

Fuchs, C. (2014) *Digital Labour and Karl Marx*. New York: Routledge.

Fuchs, C., and Sandoval, M. (2014) Digital Workers of the World Unite! A Framework for Critically Theorising and Analysing Digital Labour. *TripleC*, 12(2), 486–563.

Fumagalli, A. (2015) The Concept of Subsumption of Labour to Capital: Towards Life Subsumption in Bio-cognitive Capitalism. In E. Fisher & C. Fuchs (Eds.), *Reconsidering Value and Labour in the Digital Age* (pp. 224–245). Westminster: Palgrave Macmillan.

Hearn, A. (2010) Structuring Feeling: Web 2.0, Online Ranking and Rating, and the Digital "Reputation Economy." *Ephemera: Theory & Politics in Organization*, 10(3/4), 421–438.

Hoschchild, A. R. (1983) *The managed heart: commercialization of human feeling*. California: University of California Press.

Huws, U. (2016) *Working online, living offline: labour in the Internet Age*. Work Organisation, Labour & Globalisation, 7 (1), 1-11.

Irani, L. (2015). Difference and Dependence Among Digital Workers: The Case of Amazon Mechanical Turk. *South Atlantic Quarterly*, 114(1), 225–234.

Kosnik, A. (2013) Fandom as Free Labor. In T. Sholz (Ed.), *The Internet as Playground and Factory* (pp. 125–144). New York: Routledge.

Meil, P., & Kirov, V. (2017) *Policy Implications of Virtual Work.* London: Palgrave Macmillan. doi: 10.1007/978-3-319-52057-5.

Morini, C., and Fumagalli, A. (2010). *Life Put to Work: Towards a Life Theory of Value. Ephemera: Theory & Politics in Organization*, 10(3/4), 234–252.

Ritzer, G., and Nathan J. (2010). Production, consumption, prosumption. *Journal of Consumer Culture,* 10 (1): 13–36.

Scribano, A. (2017) *Normalization, Enjoyment & Bodies/Emotions: Argentine Sensibilities*. New York, Nova Science Publishers Inc.

Scribano, A. and Lisdero, P. (2019) *Digital Labour, Society and the Politics of Sensibilities.* Gewerbestrasse: Palgrave – MacMillan.

Smythe, D. W. (1977). Communications: Blindspot of Western Marxism. *Canadian Journal of Political and Social Theory,* 1(3), 1–27.

Terranova, T. (2013) Free Labor. In T. Scholz (Ed.), *Digital Labor. The Internet as Playground and Factory* (pp. 46–78). New York: Routledge.

Vercellone, C. (Ed.) (2006). *Capitalismo Cognitivo*. [*Cognitive Capitalism*]. Rome: Manifestolibri.

In: Emotionality of COVID-19 ISBN: 978-1-53619-534-7
Editors: M. Korstanje and S. Adrian © 2021 Nova Science Publishers, Inc.

Chapter 5

Economic, Social and Psychological Issues of Survival in the Pandemic: The Case of Russian Federation

Irina Burak [*] ***and Tatiana Razumova*** [†]
Lomonosov Moscow State University, Russian Federation

Abstract

This chapter contains the broad economic and social review of the COVID-19 consequences which Russian Federation faces today. COVID-19 epidemic update had a great impact on all spheres, people's lives had changed dramatically: many people have contracted the illness, others lost their jobs and incomes, almost all were overcome with panic. So, the main objective of the Russian Government was to rapidly develop a program of urgent response in the sphere of healthcare as well as in preventing deep negative consequences in decrease of peoples' incomes and welfare. The special measures of economic and social support were undertaken by the government towards SMEs and people under great risks of poverty. Volunteers' activities aimed at care of elderly people

[*] Corresponding Author's E-mail: irina.d.burak@mail.ru.
[†] Corresponding Author's E-mail: tatiana.razumowa@yandex.ru.

under the isolation restrictions became widely developed. To prevent the risk of contamination lots of people in different spheres were urged to work distantly, this process was supported by wide access to informational technologies and equipment and well-developed skills of specialists. Still, for many companies it was a severe challenge which required training of personnel and new management tools. During the isolation period distant professional learning was of great importance and popularity: it helped to prepare people to overcome the crisis with marketable knowledge and skills.

INTRODUCTION

The Russian Federation, together with other countries, faces serious challenges due to the pandemic. From February 2020 till April 2020 there were slowly increasing rates of infection in Russia, but then the situation became worse, so the Russian government enforced quarantine from the 30th of March. Since March 30th, restrictions were imposed on movement across the Russian border. They concerned automobile, railway, pedestrian, and river traffic, and mixed checkpoints at the border, as well as the land section of the Russian-Belarusian state border. Moreover, there were serious restrictions inside the country: on transitions between Russian regions and even between districts in big cities. A lot of attention has been paid to maintaining immediate medical services for everybody who needed them. All these efforts were implemented efficiently and successfully, and rates of contamination began to fall. But when the restrictions were lifted and people began to live their usual lives, we all faced the second wave of the Coronavirous pandemic. As of the 25th November, there are 2,162,503 Coronavirous cases in Russia, among them 1,660,419 recovery cases and 37,538 fatal outcomes. Of course, Moscow, Saint Petersburg and other big cities are the most affected (Russian Government, 2020). In such a difficult, worsening epidemiological situation, the government needs to respond quickly to new challenges and take the most effective measures to mitigate the situation and its consequences; organizations need to ensure the safest working conditions for their employees with the maximum preservation of productivity, and it is very important for citizens not to give in to panic and to observe the prescribed precautions as much as possible. That's the background we're seeing today.

SOCIO-ECONOMIC ISSUES

The first wave of the Coronavirous pandemic lasted from the second half of March 2020 till August 2020. The second wave of the pandemic, started approximately at the beginning of September 2020, slowing down the recovery of the labor market in Russia, but the number of vacancies did not decrease, as Head Hunter's research showed. According to that data, the level of competition for jobs in mid-autumn dropped slightly compared to the "before pandemic" period. On average there are six active resumes per vacancy against seven in February-March. In the second half of October the labor market experienced the second wave of the epidemic, the number of vacancies in the labor market did not fall, but the recovery trend observed since June slowed down. Thus, in October the number of vacancies published at hh.ru exceeded the figure for September by only 1%, while the annual growth is more tangible - 18%. In early November in most regions, there was a slight decrease in demand. The number of active vacancies increased only in the North-Caucasian Federal District. In early November the demand for specialists in consulting, transport and logistics, as well as in civil service, increased. The maximum decrease of demand is observed in-home staff, in tourism and hotel and restaurant businesses, as well as in the sports and beauty industries (Business Journal, 2020).

The economic situation of the Russian population during the period of self-isolation has deteriorated. According to the United Credit Bureau, in the second quarter of 2020 (April-June), working Russians lost 841 billion rubles of income. This is the equivalent of 16 million average wages. The main reason for the losses is part-time work or a reduced working week. Such measures were used by businesses to optimize costs. During the pandemic, the government financially supported certain groups, such as families with children, and subsidized entrepreneurs who did not fire employees because of the crisis. Therefore, large-scale cuts were avoided.

However, after self-isolation, the number of announcements about the sale of businesses in cities with a population of millions increased by 28% - this is indirect evidence that entrepreneurs were on the verge of bankruptcy. It can be supposed that as soon as the pandemic goes down and the government stops subsidizing businesses, small companies will start closing down and unemployment will increase (Brusentseva, Vtoraja volna koronavirusa i obshhie sny: dajdzhest trendov obshhestva № 20, 2020).

During the Coronavirous lockdown in Russia, unemployment rose by 30% on average in the regions. Many companies reduced their employees during quarantine or ceased to exist at all. Moscow, St. Petersburg and the Moscow region were the most affected by layoffs, while 3.5 million employees have been laid off since the beginning of the pandemic. According to the Russian Federal State Statistics Service (Rosstat), the total number of unemployed in the country exceeded 4.5 million in May 2020, and the unemployment rate reached a record 6.1%. In July, registered unemployment growth slowed by a third, and the market began to slowly recover after restrictive measures were lifted (Sycheva, 2020).

The social network "Odnoklassniki" and the research center "ResearchMe" conducted an online survey on women's income during the Coronavirous pandemic. The study involved 1,603 women over the age of 18. One in five women claimed they had lost their jobs during the pandemic. Most affected were the respondents between 18 and 24 years of age (30%). Among those who lost their jobs during the pandemic, about 36% have not yet found new employment. Women aged 25-34 noted that employment was hindered by the presence of a child (22%), while in the group of respondents over 45 years old the cause of difficulties in employment most mentioned was that of age (49%). According to the survey results, 61% of female respondents who worked during the pandemic experienced a decrease in their monthly income (Telegraph Agency of the Soviet Union (TASS), 2020).

The pandemic and general quarantine have confused all previous plans of employers. Some companies have started to send employees on vacation for an indefinite period and reduce their salaries, and most employers are waiting for the situation to develop and have suspended recruitment, while some continue to hire staff. According to the recruitment company Antal Russia, 12% of employers stopped recruiting employees in February and 40% in March. The share of those who planned to fill vacancies decreased from 47% to 21% during the month. 75% of companies have already reduced their staff costs due to coronavirus. 54% cancelled team retreats and teambuilding, 47% saved on travel expenses (business trips were cancelled), and 43% reduced the cost of education and training. Furthermore, 26% of respondents said they are looking for ways to avoid salary cuts and the cancellation of bonuses (Podtserob, 2020).

According to the KPMG survey "HR Actions in the Situation of the Pandemic," 49% of respondents - large companies - have already translated face-to-face interviews fully online, and 22% - partially. In the next year, 59% of companies will optimize personnel costs, 44% will switch to a new management model (flexible schedule, remote work, online recruitment), and 41% will automate personnel management processes. The study also says that after the end of the crisis, regular management practices will include the tools that had to be switched to during the epidemic: remote work (36% of respondents), online recruitment (46%) and online training (41%) (Podtserob, 2020). In this respect, Coronavirous has given a powerful impetus to cloud technologies. In the first half of the year alone the demand for them grew by 30%. Thanks to the migration to the cloud, companies working mainly in the delivery of food, FMCG goods and electronics, managed to survive organizational "overloads" associated with the transition to the "remote." While the sites of those companies, which in the old days relied on their own data centers, regularly lost profits. Quarantine and fear of infection led to strong growth in e-commerce and e-retail. Thus, according to the research center "NAFI," 67% of Russians during self-isolation ordered food and non-food products in online stores. The share of online purchases in the FMCG market almost doubled compared to 2019: from 1.9% in 2019 to 3.2% in March 2020. It is expected to grow to 4% by the end of 2020. Moreover, isolation has led to accelerated modernization of remote communication technologies in several areas at once. On the one hand, many companies have started to establish new technology solutions, which were previously considered "non-priority" to ensure synchronization of all processes outside the office, as well as to integrate chat bots and applications for the analysis of big data (Sysoev, 2020).

On the other hand, for the first time, telemedicine became a truly global trend. For example, in the first half of 2020, remote medical consultations through mobile applications and online services increased by 177% compared to the corresponding period in 2019. In response, both the development of algorithms for medical artificial intelligence (AI) and the development of AI services for the decoding of medical images have intensified (Sysoev, 2020).

The market situation has formed a "window of opportunity" for all digital segments of the economy. E-commerce, companies offering digitization business services, online video, online games and many other digital services are now growing. The field of online education is one of them. Schools, universities and kindergartens forced to switch to remote operation in an accelerated mode were generally not ready for this "new normality." Not all teachers have been able to quickly restructure the learning process "from a distance," arrange lessons and lectures in such a way as to retain students' attention and move to an individual, more flexible teaching process. Besides, not all teachers have been able to quickly adapt to new learning technologies on online platforms. Parents were also not ready for a remote format, mainly for combining work and supervising their child's learning (Sysoev, 2020). The Russian school education system was not ready for online education. The technical equipment of schools, teachers and pupils still leaves much to be desired. At the moment of urgent changes teachers did not know how to teach effectively online and could not get fast methodological and administrative support from above. It was a systemic failure which, although not officially recognized, was understood by all participants. At the same time, the Ministry of Education tried to face the truth and take quick steps to correct various processes, including involving commercial companies and platforms (Mjagkov, 2020).

Recently, together with the research group EdMarket and TalentTech, one of the largest EdTech companies in Russia "Netology-groups" has conducted a study of the online education market: in 2019 its volume amounted to 38.5 billion rubles. With “pre-quarantine” growth rates by 2023, this figure would reach 60 billion rubles. It’s worth noting that Edtech grew significantly before Coronavirous and the pandemic has only sped it up. For example, in “Foxford” - a project focused on schoolchildren - more than a million new users registered during the first week of quarantine (Spiridonov, 2020).

The free access to courses opened by many online platforms is an opportunity for mass users to at least try distance learning in its various forms. But it may take time for everyone to get used to the online format and start learning fully. The trend for digitalization of business, which has been going on for several years, but during the pandemic is more relevant than ever, affects business education as well. On the one hand, it may seem that the crisis is hitting hard on the sector of business education, making it less popular due to the worsening economic situation. But this is not true; traditionally all segments of business education, including MBA programs, are in great demand during the crisis in the market. Managers and top managers today are most eager to learn how to run a digital business: business strategy development, teamwork, management and administration, sales and marketing with a focus on digitalization. And the interest is observed in representatives of companies from all market segments, even such conservative ones as medicine and construction. And business education is ready to take into account the needs of the business, to adapt to them and offer relevant and current knowledge. Changes in the employer’s requirements for employees are based on changes in the set of competencies for certain positions. For example, to perform the functions of the head of the planning and financial department, a leading economist does not need to obtain a second higher education; in addition to the available knowledge in the field of economics and finance, it is enough for him or her to master managerial competencies. Through further professional education, the employee can fill in gaps in the required skills in a short period. In times of economic instability, employees may face the challenge of retaining them in the workplace, which is also possible through further professional education programs that will strengthen the employee's competitive position in the labor market (Razumova & Burak, 2019).

The initial increase in productivity shown by workers transferred from home to work was quickly replaced by an increase in fatigue. There were several contributing factors at once: lack of workspace, specific 'home factors' such as children, relatives or neighbors that constantly distract attention, lack of communication in the team, and excessive or minimal control by the employer. All this has become an obstacle to normal work, which for many has resulted in a loss of motivation to work. The uncertainty factor associated with the unstable economic situation and layoffs, which affected many industries, was also imposed on this. So, the spring prophecies about the "convenience" and "efficiency" of remote work were false for many people. On the contrary, we can say that today a new privilege has been formed - to work in an office at least for a few days a week. In fact, as JLL's global research shows, post-pandemic demand for office space may not be so different from recent trends. Instead, the way space is used will change. Lower occupancy levels will be compensated for by allocating more space to each workplace. Employers will pay more attention to supporting direct communications, learning and development, creativity and collaboration - the real reasons why people want to work together (Sysoev, 2020).

Sharing services are gaining popularity on the labor market, and at all levels - from simple tasks to expensive consultations. For many of those who have lost their job, but have the right skills, it becomes a way to stay afloat, and for companies a means to save money. Uberisation is not just a cab service: business in Russia uses sharing to get the expertise of highly competent specialists. Another common type of request on the sharing platform is an independent opinion. Companies focused on rapid growth are not always ready to spend time on long study and long decision-making when the issue can be resolved with independent analysis from an external expert within an hour (Bindjuk, 2020).

Because of the Coronavirous pandemic, it became more difficult for a migrant worker to come to Russia to work. According to the Ministry of Internal Affairs, in August 2020, 33.9 thousand people received work permits; a year earlier there were 82.4 thousand. According to a study by the Center for Strategic Research (CSR), 40% of companies are now experiencing labor shortages. The deficit of couriers and cab drivers is especially acute. The business is again moving employees to remote locations and the number of orders in online stores is growing. However, due to the outflow of migrants, there is no one to deliver additional orders. Many residents of the regions, who lost their jobs in the capital during the pandemic, have returned home (Brusentseva, 2020). For regional companies, who have vacancies, this is a chance to hire good specialists and implement new projects.

PSYCHOLOGICAL ISSUES

Sudden changes have now occurred in everyone's lives. They happened faster than the human mind can adapt. The overall level of fear and anxiety, which has increased significantly due to the pandemic and the global economic crisis, may lead to unwanted long-term psychological consequences, experts believe. On the one hand, the fear of a future filled with uncertainty may not only increase the already high level of anxiety but also lead to a deep depression, especially among the poor. On the other hand - for people with a genetic predisposition to some forms of obsessive-compulsive disorder (OCD) - i.e., various obsessions leading to compulsive actions - COVID-19 stress can only exacerbate OCD.

Compared to other generations, during the period of self-isolation, "zoomers" (youth aged about 11-25 years) felt the worst. Mainly, they complained about a feeling of boredom (51%), less physical activity (47%) and an increased sense of loneliness (41%). They also expressed concern about the negative impact on health due to increased screen time: 31% vs. 25% of millenniums and 14% of Gen X. The younger generation was also more likely to experience increased anxiety and stress compared to the older generation: for example, almost half of the "zoomers" said they were worried about COVID-19 (Sysoev, 2020).

Brand Analytics decided to analyze how the COVID was discussed during the year in Russia, Ukraine, Kazakhstan, Belarus, Armenia and Moldova. Where the COVID-anxiety was higher, what are the dynamics and platforms for discussion, and whether there is a correlation between the dynamics of references and the dynamics of morbidity. To understand how much the topic of Coronavirous excited people in different countries from the full flow of messages in the social media of each country, publications with mentions of COVID-19 was highlighted. Taking into account the population size, the index of "COVID-anxiety" equal to the number of mentions of the virus subject for a day for every 10 thousand of the country's population was calculated. The peak of anxiety everywhere occurred at the end of March. The greatest degree of anxiety was demonstrated by Russians and Moldovans. Inhabitants of Ukraine and Belorussia were less worried; the latter joined the discussion of COVID later than others. In Kazakhstan and Armenia, users were less actively discussing coronavirus publicly. In the central regions of Russia, residents met the second wave more calmly. The anxiety increases with the distance from the center (Cherniy, 2020).

The top 5 the most "alarming" regions look like this:

1. Magadan Region - 132 (COVID-anxiety index)
2. Chukotka Autonomous Okrug - 127
3. Republic of Crimea - 123
4. Kurgan region - 107
5. Jewish Autonomous Region - 97

The top 5 "quietest" regions were:

1. Chuvash Republic - 35
2. Kabardino-Balkarian Republic - 35
3. Pskov region - 35
4. Sakhalin Oblast – 35
5. Republic of Dagestan – 34 (Cherniy, 2020).

According to the All-Russian Public Opinion Research Center (VTsIOM) survey, 15% of Russians believed that Russia was going through the worst period of the pandemic in September 2020. Another 16% answered that all difficulties are over. But the majority (60%) is sure that hard times await them in the future. In particular, the difficulties will be related to the economic crisis. But this is not the only concern of Russians (VTsIOM, 2020).

The Public Relations Development Company (PRDC) has published a new "National Index of Concerns," a survey that shows what fears are prevalent in society. PRDC experts assess phobias by analyzing media materials and discussions on social networks. To make the rating, they use the media young index (MJng). It is calculated as a ratio of three variables: the frequency of appearance of a worrying topic in the media, its popularity in social networks and the duration of discussion of the topic. In the course of the study, PRDC analyzed 130,000 media publications and 1 million posts in social networks from June to the end of September 2020 (Brusentseva, 2020).

These are the four reasons why Russians are most worried:

- The second wave of Coronavirous (total index 353.27);
- Russia's participation in the political crisis in Belorussia (129.99);
- Dismissals and unemployment (122.06);
- Environmental pollution (63.06).

Interestingly, the first three problems are most frequently mentioned in media reports, while the climate agenda is discussed in social networks and media with equal frequency (ratio 1.09). This indicates the relevance of the topic for society and the involvement of Russians in the discussion (Brusentseva, 2020).

Due to social isolation, time spent with the family has naturally increased, and this can play an important role in the next generation of children. The fact that parents accustomed to business trips and office work have settled at home and become more flexible in structuring time can lead to a change in priorities within the family through a more balanced distribution of work and personal time. A truly comfortable family environment will result in parents being able to work more efficiently. By the way, transformations can also happen to children: although COVID-19 has further strengthened the role of technology in the life of the "Alpha generation," the virus has emphasized the value of personal communication for them (Sysoev, 2020).

According to a survey of the research company Ipsos, after the abolition of self-isolation, the level of happiness in Russia increased by 11%. This is a record figure among 27 countries in which the study was conducted. The same high value was recorded in China. Despite the sharp increase, Russia took only 18th place in the ranking of countries in terms of happiness. In first place was China, as 94% of the Chinese consider themselves happy (Ipsos, 2020).

Table 1. Level of Happiness

	Dec-11	May-13	Mar-17	Feb-18	Jun-19	Aug-20	Change since December 2011	Change since June 2019
Global Average	77%	77%	61%	70%	64%	63%	-14%	-1%
China	78%	79%	84%	85%	82%	93%	15%	11%
Netherlands						87%		
Saudi Arabia	83%	74%	75%	76%	78%	80%	-3%	2%
Canada	85%	83%	81%	81%	86%	78%	-7%	-8%
France	84%	81%	68%	77%	80%	78%	-6%	-2%
Australia	86%	84%	72%	82%	86%	77%	-9%	-9%
Great Britain	79%	81%	71%	78%	82%	76%	-3%	-6%
Sweden	80%	87%	74%	81%	75%	74%	-6%	-1%
Germany	76%	77%	71%	68%	78%	73%	-3%	-5%
Belgium	80%	80%	71%	80%	73%	71%	-9%	-2%
United States	85%	83%	80%	82%	79%	70%	-15%	-9%
Poland	75%	72%	66%	71%	71%	68%	-7%	-3%
India	89%	87%	78%	83%	77%	66%	-23%	-11%
Brazil	77%	81%	56%	73%	61%	63%	-14%	2%
Italy	73%	68%	53%	60%	57%	62%	-11%	5%
Malaysia				69%	52%	62%		10%
Turkey	89%	83%	58%	60%	53%	59%	-30%	6%
Russia	61%	62%	56%	62%	47%	58%	-3%	11%
Japan	70%	69%	62%	60%	52%	55%	-15%	3%
South Korea	71%	62%	48%	57%	54%	54%	-17%	0%
South Africa	79%	83%	59%	72%	59%	52%	-27%	-7%
Mexico	78%	80%	43%	67%	59%	46%	-32%	-13%
Hungary	43%	52%	48%	48%	50%	45%	2%	-5%
Argentina	68%	67%	48%	56%	34%	43%	-25%	9%
Spain	63%	57%	43%	53%	46%	38%	-25%	-8%
Chile			41%	71%	50%	35%		-15%
Peru			36%	54%	58%	32%		-26%

The increase in the level of happiness in Russia in the short term after the period of self-isolation can be explained by the removal of restrictions on such important universal things as meetings, personal communication, and free movement. During the period of self-isolation people have never felt their importance and value, and after the removal of restrictions a return of the lost and the feeling that the pandemic has retreated, allowed many to feel the tide of happiness in life (Ipsos, 2020).

The things that bring Russians happiness are children (59%) and relationships with a partner (56%). The feeling that their life is full of meaning was mentioned by 49% of respondents, another 45% of respondents chose good living conditions and financial well-being, and a little less - 44% - health (Ipsos, 2020).

Compared to 2019, the prevalence of happiness globally has remained nearly unchanged. It has increased by at least 5 points or more in six countries, most of all China, Russia, Malaysia, and Argentina. It has decreased by 5 points or more in 12 countries, most of all Peru, Chile, Mexico, and India (Ipsos, 2020).

POLICY ISSUES

Measures to support the economy and population have been taken in different countries of the world. The introduction of quarantine measures has a serious impact on the economies of all countries. Many kinds of activities stop at once. The production scale of many enterprises is limited. That is why the support measures are very important. Several support packages have also been approved in Russia: these are point measures to support the population and several business sectors, which we will consider in detail below.

The Government of the Russian Federation is constantly developing and taking new measures to counter the spread of new Coronavirous infection. They can be divided into two groups: social and business support measures. The first group includes:

1. Benefits for families with children. All families with children under the age of 16 received financial support, and families whose average per capita income does not exceed the minimum per capita subsistence level established in the constituent entity of the Russian Federation are entitled to monthly payments.
2. Sick leave for workers over 65 years of age. Working citizens of 65 years of age or older, observing the regime of self-isolation due to Coronavirus, who have not switched to remote work and are not on vacation, can remotely issue an electronic sick leave.
3. Support for the unemployed. Citizens who have lost their jobs will be able to apply through the portal "Work in Russia" for help in finding a job, as well as to apply for registration as unemployed and apply for unemployment benefits online. Additional payments are also granted to citizens who are dismissed and recognized as unemployed and have children.
4. Helping people with disabilities. Almost all interactions to formalize a disability and receive the corresponding allowance have been transferred online. Individual rehabilitation programs are automatically implemented without additional applications.
5. Support for employees of social institutions. Additional payments apply to those institutions that have entered quarantine - that is, where employees worked for at least 14 days inside the institution to minimize the risk of infection of citizens living there.
6. Support of employees and volunteers. Special payments are made to employees of state and non-state organizations and volunteers who have accepted accompanying and temporary accommodation, including temporary care, disabled persons, older citizens, orphans and children without parental care, social service organizations and orphanages.
7. Assistance to tourists. Citizens who have planned a trip from the beginning of the restrictive measures until June 1, 2020 will be able to receive a refund for a disrupted trip. In case of cancellation of a flight abroad, which should take place during the period of prohibition of international air travel, the passenger will be

refunded the full amount for the ticket. Besides, there is an organized return of Russian citizens from abroad. For all who find themselves abroad and are unable to return to Russia due to the spread of new Coronavirus infection, the necessary social support is provided.

8. Extension of documents. Passports and driver's licenses that have expired or expire between February 1 and July 15, 2020, inclusive, are considered valid.
9. Credit vacation. This is a grace period for possible reduction or suspension of regular payments on the loan for up to 6 months. They are granted to citizens who have difficulties with payments on loans or credits, if their income for the month preceding the date of application, decreased by at least 30% compared with the average monthly income in 2019.
10. Moratorium on payment of penalties for housing and communal services. It is forbidden to levy penalties for late or incomplete payment for housing, utilities and repairs. It is also prohibited to limit the provision of utilities in case of their late payment by citizens.
11. Monitoring of essential goods. In order to prevent the spread of new coronavirus infection in Russia, a list of non-food items of prime necessity and rapid monitoring of their availability in trade organizations was compiled so that there would not be a shortage of these items. The list of essential goods includes disinfectants and personal protective equipment, hygiene supplies and detergents, baby products, pet food, various fuels, candles, and matches. State authorities of the subjects of the Russian Federation have the right to make changes in the list of non-food items of prime necessity at the regional level based on the sanitary and epidemiological situation in the region.
12. Sale of medicines online. Medicines released without prescription can be purchased through the Internet with home delivery. It is not possible to buy prescription drugs, as well as over-the-counter drugs, narcotic and psychotropic drugs, alcohol-containing drugs

with a volume fraction of ethyl alcohol exceeding 25% via the Internet (Russian Government, 2020).

The second group contains:

1. Bankruptcy moratorium. Acceptance of creditor bankruptcy applications from creditors is suspended. The courts also suspend proceedings in accepted cases where bankruptcy proceedings have not yet commenced. The debtor is relieved of the obligation to go to court if there are signs of bankruptcy, but the right to do so remains.
2. A moratorium on business audits. Suspends field audits of small and medium-sized businesses. All licenses and permits are automatically renewed for six months. Only unscheduled inspections are preserved, the basis for which is harm to life and health of citizens, the emergence of emergencies of a natural and man-made character.
3. Credit vacation for business. Entrepreneurs can get a grace period on the loan for 6 months, as well as count on reducing the amount of deferred debt due to federal subsidies for banks, if the credit organization participates in the program of the Ministry of Economic Development. This measure applies to SMEs working in the most affected areas: air and road transport, tourism, the hotel business, catering, culture, entertainment and leisure (including cinemas, museums and zoos), physical education and sports, conferences and exhibitions, consumer services to the public, dental practice, additional education, and retail trade in non-food products.
4. Interest-free loans for salaries. Large, medium and small businesses, as well as individual entrepreneurs from the most affected industries, can take an interest-free loan from the bank for six months to pay salaries to employees. Credits for small and micro businesses will be provided by the bank, taking into account

the main and additional OKVED. For large and medium-sized companies - only the main.

5. Decrease in insurance premiums. For organizations and private entrepreneurs included in the Single Register of SMEs, the total amount of insurance premiums is reduced from 30% to 15%. The rate of contributions to the Pension Fund of Russia will be 10%, to the Federal Compulsory Medical Insurance Fund - 5%. Contributions to the Social Insurance Fund (for disability and maternity) are not paid.
6. Tax vacations. This means that almost all taxes are deferred for companies in the ten industries most affected by the epidemic and part of the taxes for all other entrepreneurs.
7. Postponement of rent payments. Delayed payment of rents applies to state, municipal and private property.
8. Assistance to exporters. The Russian Export Center provides businesspeople with targeted consultations taking into account the situation in the industry and the specifics of the enterprise. The operational headquarters of the Russian Export Center helps solve logistics problems and obtain financial support in connection with emerging cash gaps, assists in concluding new export deals and advises on a wide range of issues in the sphere of certification, subsidies, cooperation with customs authorities, etc.
9. Non-refundable subsidies. Small and medium enterprises from 11 affected industries can benefit from direct financial support from the state. Entrepreneurs can receive an amount equal to the established minimum wage per employee.
10. Extension of licenses. If a company is engaged in licensed activities, there is no need to renew licenses in 2020 - many licenses are automatically renewed for one year.
11. Support for systemically important enterprises. System forming enterprises are companies that have a significant impact on the development of the country's economy, provide the greatest employment in their industries and are the largest taxpayers. The government has developed several special measures for system-

forming enterprises: preferential credits for replenishment of working capital and maintenance of employment, special conditions for obtaining deferral or installment payments for some tax payments with payment deadlines in 2020, credits at a preferential rate can be obtained by subsidiaries of system-forming enterprises, as well as their parent companies. Besides, systemically important companies that are at special risk can also apply for subsidies to reimburse production, work and service costs and government guarantees necessary to restructure existing loans or issue new loans and bond issues.

12. Non-performing loans. Such loans may be claimed by enterprises from affected industries, as well as socially oriented non-profit organizations. For enterprises that retain at least 90% of their employees, the loan will be written off along with interest - the state will pay the entire amount. If at least 80% of employees remain on the staff, the entrepreneur will have to repay only half of the loan and the interest on it (Russian Government, 2020).

Thus, we see that we are talking about supporting the population and business through a softer monetary policy, accompanied by extensive budget guarantees, which reduce the risks of bank lending. It should be noted that the measures taken by the Russian government have helped the population and business to survive difficult times, as well as kept the country's economy from collapse, preventing a sharp downturn.

VOLUNTEER ISSUES

Within the framework of the All-Russian action of mutual assistance during the Coronavirus Pandemic "My Vmeste," volunteers help elderly people in the delivery of products, medicines and necessities, they also perform such functions as psychological and legal advice, online assistance, and volunteers with specialized education help in medical organizations. The target audience for assistance comprises elderly people and citizens with low mobility (My Vmeste, 2020). Appeals are accepted twenty-four hours a day on a "hot line." There are four main volunteer focus areas:

1. Buying and delivering products, medicines and essential commodities. People who are now at home in self-isolation due to Coronavirus need assistance in buying and delivering products, medicines and household goods. Volunteers purchase everything they need and bring it to beneficiaries observing all safety precautions.
2. Assistance with medical organizations. Due to the high load on medical staff, assistance in patient care, manipulation, document management and patient routing is required. Volunteers are distributed according to their specialization. Non-medical assistance in this area can also be joined by those who do not have a medical education.
3. Providing psychological assistance. Due to the wide spread of various information about Coronavirus infection, people are not always able to perceive it adequately, and there are stressful reactions. Volunteers with appropriate training provide psychological support to people by telephone and text consultation. To become a volunteer in this area, individuals need an education in psychology.
4. Help in call centers. Patients with a mild course of the new coronavirus infection are given outpatient treatment. Volunteers make calls to these patients using prepared scripts to monitor the dynamics of their condition and refer them to the doctor's surgery if necessary. Volunteers also respond to citizens' questions about the coronavirus, talk about its prevention and diagnosis, report the results of tests, and pass on necessary information. General volunteers and volunteers with medical education can work in this area (My Vmeste, 2020).

Each volunteer must take a distance learning course on the following topics:

- Hygienic norms for volunteers;
- Mechanism of providing volunteer assistance to elderly people;
- The specifics of interaction with elderly people;
- The actions of volunteers in emergency and non-standard situations (My Vmeste, 2020).

After that, they will receive a face-to-face briefing on safety at the headquarters in groups (up to 20 people) or individually. Then they receive an accreditation badge and admission to work, after which they undergo a check-in procedure before starting work: temperature measurement, safety briefing and receiving individual safety kits (My Vmeste, 2020).

To avoid cases of fraud, applicants are informed about the identity of the real volunteers:

- Volunteers wear a special badge and a passport.
- Volunteers are provided with personal protective equipment: a disposable medical mask, gloves and antiseptics.
- Volunteers do not enter the apartment/house.
- The volunteer knows the beneficiary's application number and must inform him/her at the beginning of communication.
- You can check the identity of each volunteer by contacting the regional volunteer organization (My Vmeste, 2020).

This is the largest, but not the only, action of mutual aid in Russia that appeared during the epidemic. Obviously, in such a difficult period, the main pressure falls on medical personnel, who also need support, including of a moral kind. For example, in Blagoveshchensk there is an action "Doctors are our heroes," where the city entrepreneurs collect gifts for medical workers to support them during the pandemic. They buy medical hand creams, moisturizing facial masks, honey and other sweets, which they put into gift sets and give to doctors who work with patients with

COVID-19. Gifts are bought at the expense of entrepreneurs and citizens who care about them. Businesspeople also donated fruit and fresh baked goods to the staff of the emergency station and Blagoveshchensk city hospital. The initiative group plans to form gifts for medical workers from hospitals in the region. The coaches and sportsmen of "Mashina" club in Blagoveshchensk help doctors unload medicines and furniture, which were transported from one medical institution to another to equip infectious diseases hospitals (My Vmeste, 2020).

CONCLUSION

Nowadays it is obvious that such a great pandemic will have a long-lasting and even controversial effect on all spheres of people's lives. And its consequences are highly dependent on the expediency and efficiency of specific measures undertaken by the government and peoples' economic and social behavior. Of course, the Coronavirus pandemic has such a huge scale that preventing and defeating it cannot be an objective of each country in particular. There must be a strong collaboration between countries, at least between those who have common frontiers.

REFERENCES

Bindjuk I. Konsul'tacija na $1,5 tys. v chas: kak rabotaet shering jekspertizy v Rossii // *RBC Trends. - 2020.* – Available at https://trends.rbc.ru/trends/sharing/5f6b5c5f9a7947f51dd10144.

Brusentseva E. Trevozhnye rossijane i nehvatka rabochih ruk: dajdzhest trendov obshhestva № 21 // *RBC Trends. - 2020.* - Available at https://trends.rbc.ru/trends/social/5f92f0859a79477569f4b4fe.

Brusentseva E. Vtoraja volna koronavirusa i obshhie sny: dajdzhest trendov obshhestva № 20 // *RBC Trends.* - 2020. - Available at https://trends.rbc.ru/trends/social/5f89d7309a7947e11c7439cd.

Business Journal Volna Pandemii Zamedlila Vosstanovlenie Rynka Truda // *Federal Business Journal*. - November 2020. - Available at https://business-magazine.online/fn_44396.html.

Cherniy V. Social Media Alert Covid Index in 2020: Russia, Ukraine, Kazakhstan, Belarus, Armenia, Moldova. "Is there a second wave of discussions? // *Brand Analytics*. - October 2020. - Available at https://br-analytics.ru/blog/index-covid-social-media/.

Grigoryev L., Pavlyushina V., Muzychenko E. *The fall into 2020 recession*… [Journal]// Voprosy Ekonomiki, 2020, No. 5, pp. 5—24.

Ipsos GLOBAL HAPPINESS 2020. *What Makes People Happy in the Age of COVID*-19 [Report]. - New York : Ipsos, 2020.

Mjagkov M. "Eshhe ne gotovy k onlajn-obrazovaniju." Chto zhdet shkoly posle COVID-19 // *RBC Trends. - 2020*. - Available at https://trends.rbc.ru/trends/education/5ecb8f919a794709d4d92e53. ["Not ready for online education yet." What awaits school after COVID-19]

My Vmeste Kak volontery i biznes Priamur'ja pomogajut vracham goroda // *My Vmeste. - November 2020*. - Available at https://мывместе2020.рф/news/tpost/ftn6eummn1-kak-volonteri-i-biznes-priamurya-pomogay. [We Are Together How Priamur's volunteers and business help city doctors]

My Vmeste O funktsionale volonterov // *My Vmeste. - 2020*. - Available at https://мывместе2020.рф/volunteers. [We Are Together About the functionality of volunteers]

Podtserob M. *Kak pandemija povlijala na rossijskij rynok truda // Vedomosti*. - April 2020. - Available at https://www.vedomosti.ru/management/articles/2020/04/01/826854-kak-pandemiya-rinok-truda. [How the pandemic affected the Russian labor market]

Razumova T., Burak I. Alternative approaches to determining costs and benefits of further professional education [Journal] // *3rd International e-Conference on Studies in Humanities and Social Sciences*. - 2019. - p. 13-23.

Russian Government Measures for business support // *Stop Coronavirus*. - *2020*. - Available at https://стопкоронавирус.рф/what-to-do/business/.

Russian Government Operativnye dannye // *Stop Coronavirus. - 2020.* - Available at https://стопкоронавирус.рф.

Russian Government Social Measures // *Stop Coronavirus. - 2020.* - Available at https://стопкоронавирус.рф/what-is-done/social-measures/.

Spiridonov M. *How online education will change in the context of the pandemic // RBC.* - 2020. - Available at https://trends.rbc.ru/trends/education/5e9597339a79473072c3e718.

Sycheva I. *Kak pandemija povlijala na rynok truda v Rossii // Pravmir.* - July 2020. - https://www.pravmir.ru/kak-pandemiya-povliyala-na-rynok-truda-v-rossii-infografika/. [*How the pandemic affected the labor market in Russia*]

Sysoev T. 12 *Glavnyh posledstvij COVID-19 dlja nashego obshhestva // RBC Trends. - 2020.* - Available at https://trends.rbc.ru/trends/social/5fa195429a794721ab1f7d29. [*The main consequences of COVID-19 for our society*]

Telegraph Agency of Soviet Union (TASS) *Opros: kazhdaja pjataja zhenshhina zajavila o potere raboty vo vremja pandemii // TASS.RU.* - November 2020. - Available at https://tass.ru/obschestvo/10057075. [*Poll: 1 in 5 women said they lost their jobs during a pandemic*]

VTsIOM *Social'noe samochuvstvie rossijan: monitoring // VTsIOM. - October 2020.* - Available at https://wciom.ru/analytical-reviews/analiticheskii-obzor/soczialnoe-samochuvstvie-rossiyan-monitoring. [*Russian social self-esteem: monitoring*]

In: Emotionality of COVID-19 ISBN: 978-1-53619-534-7
Editors: M. Korstanje and S. Adrian © 2021 Nova Science Publishers, Inc.

Chapter 6

LONG LIVE TO THE URBAN FLESH

Fabio La Rocca*

LEIRIS (Researcher center of social imaginary),
University Paul-Valéry Montpellier 3, France

Panic on the streets of London
Panic on the streets of Birmingham
I wonder to myself
Could life ever be sane again?
The leeds side-streets that you slip down
I wonder to myself
Hopes may rise on the Grasmere
But honey pie, you're not safe here
So you run down
To the safety of the town
The Smiths – Panic (1987).

* Corresponding Author's E-mail: fabio.la-rocca@univ-montp3.fr.

ABSTRACT

In the present chapter we bring some reflection about changes of the current reconfigured urban space and the orientation of a revaluated vision of ecosophy with some specific elements of the ambiance that we can observe in the daily experience. With this structure, we build in our way a kind of sensible thought to elucidate a vision of some forms of urban social dimension. Our intention in this hot-debate aims to show some fragments constructing a particular vision of the spirit of the time in order to analyze the actual socio-urban dimension. In this perspective, will bring together some goals as the illustration of the actual city, the experience in the post COVID-19 situation, the idea of proximity, the new vision of ecological sensibility, where each of them encloses other peculiars aspects of our experience of the social urban world.

Keywords: Urbanity, emotions, pandemic, COVID-19, ecosophy

INTRODUCTION

How to think the city and its spaces in the actual social situation? We assist in a renewal of the approach of the way to live in urban space and the changes in the lifestyle. Is the city in crisis? It is dead? What is its future?

The explosion of the epidemic situation has generated a particular condition in the whole world where the imposition of 'social distancing' and the political interventions about the virus Covid 19 have transformed the face of the city. One of the first impressions is that we witness a materialisation of post-apocalyptical imaginary, the catastrophic dimension of urban space where the persons disappear and the city becomes empty of social life. This is a sort of imaginary to live on new ruins of an actual social world where all the images that circulate on social media, on tv, web or journals, exhibit the empty cities as we lived in a kind of science-fiction dimension: Into the void.

Despite all, the first global lockdown shows us a 'particular beauty' of the cities: it's a paradox maybe, but strangely all the images that we have consumed can be considered as 'the unsettling beauty' or a 'sadness beauty' of global cities. The images of empty cities that we observed, like Time Square in New York that is usually a pulsing heart, or California Street in San Francisco without the full dimension of tram and cars, the alleys of Venice, Plaza Mayor in Madrid, Ponte Vecchio in Florence, Champs Élysées in Paris, habitually places of the crowd and animated temporalities like many other examples. This gives us the feeling that the city without the human is more romantic, attractive, scenic! Everyone in front of these images can have the impression of this 'strange beauty.'

Our intention in this reflection, is to show some aspects or better some fragments constructing a particular vision of the spirit of the time in order to analyze the actual socio-urban dimension. The fragments are like images of thinking, as the work of Walter Benjamin teaches us, to illustrate the signs of our present and re-think our time. In this perspective, will bring together some goals as the illustration of the actual city, the experience in the Covid situation, the idea of proximity, the new vision of ecological sensibility, where each of them encloses other peculiars aspects of our experience of the social urban world. In the first step, we clarify the image of the city through the effect of the pandemic situation and after concentrate the reflection about how the Covid affects our life in the urban and the interior dimension with the particular effect of digital experience. After that, the discussion will be oriented towards the notion of proximity and the semiotic changes of the current reconfigured urban space and the orientation of a revaluated vision of ecosophy with some specific elements of the ambiance that we can observe in the daily experience. With this structure, we build in our way a kind of sensible thought to elucidate a vision of some forms of urban social dimension.

Short Debate: The City

The desert city, the phantom city, or the silent city where one can just listen to the sound of nature. These are the impressions of a fascinating atmosphere where the calm dominates transforming the city into a unique historical moment. We can witness this show during a digital promenade on Instagram where is possible to rediscover the splendor of the city. This illustrates a kind of impossible dream of seeing the beauty of the landscape without traffic, pollution, noises… The pandemic is affecting the emotional aspect of the images that circulate as conversational moments of daily life shared by the internauts (or netizen). They create a mosaic of this kind of landmark proving the world as a post-apocalyptic appearance. During this period, we have been spectators of external life from the interior. Our windows represent a porosity instrument, a medium to look at this spectacular desert. At the same time all the web's windows permitting us to circumnavigate all over the city of the globe to assist at this world in ruins. In this perspective, we can think, in reference to the theory of Walter Benjamin, at a compenetrating of spaces. That would be a duality where the urban space has a texture of an image like a new kind of phantasmagoria. It would allow us to dream, from the windows, the external urban life. This particular porosity represents an allegoric form of presence with an emphasis on emotions and feelings. Emotions must be understood as a social language, a collective expression, in the perspective of Marcel Mauss (1921). In our reflection, we can see how the extension of the interior of our apartments during the lockdown was exteriorized from the window to create a social manifestation of an emotional tribality (Maffesoli, 1988). It's an emotional resonance that the people create with this kind of 'sociology of balconies.' It became an expression to this extension from inside to outside, the intimacy became extremity (*extimité*) according to the analysis of the French psychiatric Serge Tisseron. Our balconies and windows, from Paris to Naples, from New York to Barcelona, etc., testified this desire to make visible the aspects of our social existence without the possibility to be on the street. It gave the possibility to live the street through the lockdown. We can conceive them as an 'opening on the world' (Teyssot, 2009) or also as an instrument of political act. Show drawing of children, clapping, sing together as a kind of flash mob, the music on high volume are some actions that people organize from this particular space, the balcony, became for a special period the 'new street.'

This special emotional moment describes an imaginary of 'cultural apocalypse,' using here a terminology of the Italian anthropologist Ernesto Di Martino (1977), that indicates a relevant change transforming the entire community of people. The apocalypse means the end of a paradigm and its cultural organization that generate the production of a new kind of behavior, thought and interests. Each epoch can have its 'end of a world' that signifies a deeper social change and, in our reflection, an actual reconfiguration of urban life. The question, following Di Martino, is about the 'how.' In our consideration how is or must be the human in the city and this 'how' represents an ontological question of the presence and the way to be in the world and renovate it through different forms. How is the way to be in the social world and in the urban dimension in this particular *zeitgeist*? The approach of Georg Simmel concerning the idea of sociology as *nova scienza* (a notion used by Gianbattista Vico) is relevant in this consideration. Reality isn't static but always in movement and the same goes for the city and its urban atmospheres. So, we must observe this reality in movement and try to put in evidence some forms, some essential characters. In this direction the modalities we inhabit the world are in relation to the urban sphere. In this case, the balcony assumes a significant dimension of social interrelation fusing with the digital space to create a fortification of the social connection.

THE COVID-19 AND THE EXPERIENCE

COVID-19 instils emotional affectivity of the human action also developed via the web life's experience creating. Therefore, it becomes an expressive space, or a 'grammar of experience' (Goffman, 1991) made possible through the urban photos shared by the citizens to show the reality of the present city. It shows a city of ghosts lived by images that remind us of an imaginary post-apocalyptic. This is carried by science fiction or from the narration by tv-series and cinema that absorb reality in a kind of melancholic feeling. This can be the logic that constructs a type of presentation of the vestiges of our social dimension. They are almost like a romantic scene suggesting, additionally, a scenario of quietness where the city became a postcard. But at the same time, this sad beauty is the sign of the time dominated by the 'a-social' dimension of the pandemic. The city struggles with the effect of reciprocity interaction and its fundamental quality: the instrument to be present, to inhabit the world. In fact, the relation of individual/urban space is one of the primary meanings of the way to inhabit the world. The destruction of social relations with the spacing means, at the same time, the ruination of the urban social dimension with the lockdown factor that isolates people inside, thus developing an electronic social construction of reality.

The electronic space, lived in the sharing life of emotions, show us the potentiality of the digital windows creating a conceivable manner to stay together and animate the world. The outside without human beings seems something different. Many opinions put the accent on the possibility to appreciate the beauty of the urban landscape, the soundscape of the urban structure with the absence of noises, the flowering of nature. This makes us think about the place of humans. Today, many discourses arguments about 'how' to think the city of tomorrow with the resilience, the co-construction with nature or simply a more ecological city. But at the same time, we can perceive the intensity of technological control with drones, cameras, new apps and militarization generating contemporary anxiety by surveillance.

So, how to think the actual transformation and of social life through the urban space? (Re) think the urban space pay attention to dissimilar elements but, succinctly, suggest that the urban body is a part of us, an extension of the human body. The new settlement and frequent of the street are synonymous of an intensity to be together. The street is a magma, a social glue indicating societal energy that must never die. The importance of the street for the construction of social reality means to revoke the duality individual/urban space as an evident element of vitalism. Life is also synonymous of the street and urban sections where the Being is externalized as an ontological dimension. The open windows with the sound of music from inside that invade the street, for example, was one of the modalities or better a tactic, following the idea of the 'invention of daily life' in Michel de Certeau (1981). It marks a presence, to animate the outside and construct an emotional atmosphere shared with the others.

We know how emotions are important to the structure of daily life. Urbanity is also designed from this point because emotions participate in the creation of urban ambience as a sensorial impact on the human and urban spaces. The emotions can be considerate, through the senses of course, as an interface between the urbanity and the individuals configuring our environment and the way to be in this environment. Urbanity must be considered not only for the simple functions or materiality but it is necessary to put attention on the 'immateriality' i.e., the way we feel the urbanity. We can also talk about sensations, sentiments that allow a perception of the city. It would compose an imaginary of emotional spaces shared by the individuals and, in this direction, we assist to particular manners to do, to be in the space considering also the porosity inside/outside.

The spatial dimension acquires new sensorial forms as consequences to the reconfiguration of the space to manage the pandemic situation. We can perceive in the urban panorama new signs and symbols that the individuals must recognize in its visual sensitivity as a kind of new alphabetization of spatial semiotic. The predominating of visuality is one of the keys of lectures to approach the urbanity and because it's one of the most stimulated senses and our eyes must decrypt many stimuli to read the city as a text. The various signs and symbols became a language for us and all the transformations change the inter-sensorial mode to be in the space developing as well the social reality in the urban configuration. In this phase, we can assist in a reorganisation of space through new codes to decipher and interpret. In this layout, we can say that there is a new alphabetisation because we must reorganize our visual perception. It is possible to apprehend a new symbolic language that redefines our urban social life in the optic to observe the relations between social comportment and urban forms. One can talk about altered architectonic affecting new categories of open and enclosed spaces where generate different settlements of distance.

The Notion of Proximity

Proximity is within a re-arrangement of presence where demarcations, limits, restrictions transform our spaces of 'contacts,' often generating a crisis of presence. In fact, one of the first appearances was to desert urban life with many places closed. It is impossible to be lived because the settlement was the non-contact and the inside private space was the 'safe' universe. The non-contact or more common the 'social distance,' influences and re-defined the practice of the social urban space. New sensorial orientations are also the significance of the practice that the individual must interiorise concerning the multiple marks on the ground. These marks proliferate actually in our cities on the sidewalk or inside the malls, schools, markets, shops, etc. The sensorial attitude is characterized by the signals directing our glance, signs and symbols of new social parameters to be in the space. They remind to manners to apply with the calculation of distance, use of masks, put the gel, wash your hands, etc. This is the visual symbolic panorama of the actual urban situation. Individuals are confronted to recognize some signs incarnate in the new dimension of architecture and urbanism. This also means a new perspective of the significance of something that changes our mental, corporal and emotional feeling within the city. An epochal question that arises in a complex dimension with a phenomenological topic where the city must answer with a proposition of mutations in conformity with the distinctive situation. In this condition, the urban and architectural factors are considered as an illustration of inhabited spaces. It has a direct impact on forms of perception of external and interior lived spaces because are a prolongation of the individual and the evident manifestation of social behaviours with a determinate influence on lived experience.

There is a relation between the natural space and the anthropized space that configures the social landscape. It's a typology of the aesthetical process of architecture and spatial dimensions as a predisposition to lived experience. It must assume a disposition to the strategy of 'transformability' of the city and, consequently, human nature. Many questions and interrogations of possible changes and directions are stipulated where the urban and social dimensions must answer for a 'better' future! The problem is that we put many attentions on the future and we forget the present, the lived experience in the *hic et nunc* of our situation. The impression is that people need urban places to be present in the world. This is because there is a concatenation, a vitality of forms between human being and urban spaces. We see that the reaction of people after the confinement was the invasions of the street, the pleasure to be on terraces of bars, restaurants, coffees that means, simply, a manifestation of social life presence. The pandemic situation creates a kind of annihilation of urban atmosphere generating mutations of sensations. This does not mean that social vitalism is gone! But just a kind of an 'adaptation to the situation,' a famous theorem of William Isaac Thomas, where people 'do with' (as a strategy of daily life in Michel de Certeau theory and Michel Maffesoli idea of real). This 'do with' is also accommodation, adjustment, where people readapt its manners to respond to a social situation.

THE ECOLOGY RE-IMAGINED

The key can be to reinvent new codes where the space is hybrid with contamination and not just a simple function. It is similar to 'open urbanism' proposed by the reflection of Richard Sennet, in some recent interviews, with a flexible environment and the proposition of porosity to redefine the structure and manners. The problem is to think of a way to inhabit, the way we use the physical environment and how the behaviour can be adequate. One of the most recurrent opportunities to adapt the social life is the pregnancy of a green attitude. In our reflection, it would be better for the emphasis on the eco-sophycal perspective to understand the pregnancy on the sensible and the collective way to inhabit. The ecosophy for the French philosopher Félix Guattari (2013) is an articulation between nature or environment, social relations and subjectivity. In our opinion, this synergy influences urbanity and the architecture and the way to live in the urban and social geography and represents a specific relation of an ontology of actual dimensions. Ontologically the need for 'nature,' also illustrated by the important contribution of the theory of Augustin Berque, is integrated into the connection that the human being has with its environment and *milieu*. It is an 'onto-geographical' relation (Berque, 2000) that redefines the attention of nature as the interaction between the individuals and space. The way we are interconnected to the urban social environment is also characterized by the way to feel through the sensible perception that generates a particular ambience. This produces a spatial experience and way to inhabit. The discussion about 'green' today is very common. Nevertheless, our intention isn't an ideological reflection but a consideration of a relation with the contest where we live to re-build the social reality. The city, in this direction, represents a significant element to think about the aesthetic of ecosophical paradigm from the recreative forms to inhabit. This signifies a new creation of the sense of urbanology that put the attention on the knowledge of the city and its lived spaces. The ecosophy must be thanked, following the proposition of Maffesoli (2010) as a way to be in the world.

The idea of Guattari was also to think the hypothesis of ecology as a mode to re-invent new manners to be in the world and new forms of sociality. The ecosophical sensibility can be a societal transformation with a particular highlighting on the relational ethic. This can be in consonance with the proposition of Arne Næss (2008) about a relational ontology where all the forms of life are interdependent. This interdependence can be based on some attention about architectural forms and the transformation of the inhabited landscape, where the technology has a big impact on the contribution of the mutations. The rhythm of actual urbanology is structured by the immersion in a relation between technique, culture and technology. Often the perception, when we think to the association urbanity and technology, is something similar to a dystopic sensation (i.e., a type of *black mirror* scenario[1]). Technology is control of urban space and during the pandemic period, we have assisted to a 'dronization' of the territory. This fed the idea of an immersive control also structured by some apps of our smartphone and QR codes to verify the displacement of people

[1] The reference, of course, is to the British dystopian series *Black Mirror* created by Charlie Brooker.

in the epoch where we transform ourselves into simple data... Examples, among others, confirming a political strategy of control, an increase of surveillance as the progress of a new *Big Brother watching us*!

We don't have the intention to enter here in this argument that also generates many reactions about neo-liberalism and the asphyxia of terror provoked by the pandemic that struggles our social reality through the social distance and all the gestures we must apply. But we know that the human being needs contacts and, in this situation, new technology is also used to create forms of socialization (and in our opinion isn't a novelty), forming a digital society where the union between the Net and the lived spaces are a common fact. The city is more eco-systemic where the informatics architecture transforms the relation creating a rhizomatic experienced established on the connectivity. This generates hybridism of experiences and vital flux. In the optic of thought proposed by Massimo Di Felice (2010; 2012), we are in a biosphere defined like an 'info-material' where the individual is in interaction with nature through media prothesis creating an 'atopic connection.' For Di Felice, the informatics architecture based on the Net and with interactive and connective ecology produces another vision of the ecology that isn't a simple idea of the environment. On the contrary, it is a complex union of networks composing a new form to inhabit the world that we can call cohabitation. This generates at the same time a new version of a 'poetics of the space.' Poetic that the famous French philosopher Gaston Bachelard (1957) explained like a sensible phenomenology of the space and the instantaneity of lived experience. Urban spatiality is a coincidence with the existential spatiality.

In this direction, we must think that the interconnection of the physical environment with the social atmosphere and the human actions and the environment represent our surroundings. Well, it is obvious that one of the questions of our times is the requalification of the urbanity with special attention of the ecosophy and not simple ecology. A requalification that also concerns the life-style and the production of new spatiality where is possible to re-enchant the urban ecosystem. In this illustration, the biophilia seems to be a tendency of contemporary life. It represents a connection with nature and also a kind of well-being generating some specific configurations in an urban atmosphere. Our relation to nature products this 'biophilic city' where the cohabitation and the nature can be factors of social cohesion. In the optic of urban planning and metropolitan design, the empathy with nature is a topic that recreates the social urban space. The design conception of urban spaces, in fact, put the focus on biodiversity through the conception of spaces that sensitize the ecosophical values producing, in this way, a reciprocal relationship between human, nature and urbanity. We can also understand the vegetal design trying to engender well-being in urban dimensions as a strategy of social reconstruction of reality.

The vegetal design transforms our imaginary of nature creating a valorization of this effect and an urban emotionality linked to the 'vegetalization' of daily life experience. The idea of biophilia is one of the tendencies to regenerate our urban body. This can produce a straightening of social ties where space plays a vital role. The presence of nature, a strategy more and more current in the discussion of the city 'post-covid,' must be read like the creation of sensible ambience that influences the sensorial perception of the citizen and creates a kind of pleasantness. We can feel more and more in all the cities and for the human body, this necessity of green. In fact, one of the consequences of the lockdown was the escape from the metropolis and the refuge in green spaces outside from urbanity (that means in our opinion the danger to destruction the countryside). For this reason, some actual project – that we can also define as a projection of a sci-fi imaginary –, concentrates the attention on the 'post-covid city' as the eco-district thanked in the perspective of a self-sufficient city.

For instance, we can refer to the project in China by the Spanish architect Vicente Guallart. Its proposition of 'self-sufficient city" is a response to the climate catastrophe and to the covid crisis. It can generate new forms of architecture and lifestyle with the integration of porosity. This is also the idea of the theorization of the concept 'the 15-minute city' idealized by Carlos Moreno, one of the pioneers of the 'Smart City,' as an urban design approach to ameliorate the quality of life. This is done by creating cities where all the residents can reach everything they need within 15 minutes by bike, public transports, walk. A 'no-car city' we could say, following the dream of the current Paris Mayor Anne Hidalgo that is one of the most enthusiastic supporters of this kind of city in her proposition to transform the *City of Light*. For Moreno (2020), the object is the city of proximity with a massive network of places redefining the lifetime, a redefinition of the idea of city form that must overlook the 'world-city.' We must understand the mutations and risks of climatic change, new pandemic and the extreme forms of neo-liberalism and savage capitalism that smashed the social reality.

The project of Guallart and the idea of Moreno are conceptions of the mutation provoked by the actual crisis. They offer a proposition of a lifetime harmony where, again, the porosity as an extension is one of the keys. There are also many other suggestions where the individual has a central place and can contribute. We think to the 'makers' for example, to the reconfiguration of urban social life. For us, the mutation is also an occasion to humanize spaces through nature, reintegrate green strategies. The mutation is not just some interesting ideas and actualization of interventions (green architecture, shared gardens, vegetal wall…) but rather ontological and paradigmatic. This means rethinking the urbanity from 'natural green' creation as integration in the life-style. This also adds a poetic and sensible dimension as the complement of the re-signification of urban social life as a possibility to think all this arrangement as facilitation of eco-systems in an organic city to think like a body with its flesh, skin, organs. This is, at the same time, a mode to actualize the transformation of urbanity and the renewal of the urban panorama where the vegetation of lived spaces became a style that proliferates.

This must be imagined as an answer to the nervous intensification of life that showed Georg Simmel (1903) as the effect on the metropolitan cities. The ecosophy of the urban space, following the thought of Simmel, can be a way to forge the psychology of the urban and the way to think. For this reason, all the 'natural' conception are emblems of an eco-societal stabilisation of actual metropolis with the scope to transmute the manners to live-together.

We can propose the idea of an 'organi-city' like an inclination to the modes to edify the human and urban habitat by the sensible mutation of the ambience. It offers a social harmony between human and environment where, for the ecosophical perspective, the man and the world are aspects of the same reality. And in this reality often we listen to discussions about the concept very common and popular like the resilience with the proposition of a 'resilient city' as a strategy of urban regeneration. This that signifies adequacy to the spirit of the time to develop the community capacity of a way to inhabit-together as a mode to be in the world; adaptation of a new form of urban life with an emergency of socio-aesthetical solidarity. But the 'resilient city' is often thanked as models of planning of risks and vulnerability of society. This is more 'collapsologycal' (another popular concept that invades our daily life with the proliferation of opinions and catastrophic analysis).

In our intention, associating to resilience the *reliance* (a way to be linked), we try to think to a process where the *homo urbanus* is connected to the *milieu* in its organic experience where the actions are a synergy of eco-social-urban well-being. In this sensibility, we can feel the tonality with spaces through sensible experience where the individuals adapt the way to be with the environment. Being in tonality in a sensible and effective way is a reflection about the importance of ambience. It also reflects the *Stimmung* that in Heidegger *Sein und Zeit* is a way to have access to being there, a manifestation of being revealing a *das Gestimmtstein* that means 'to be-intoned.' The intonation is a harmonic disposition that, in a reflection about the actual reality of the city, can be in relation to nature, to the ecosophical essence.

CONCLUSION

After further discussion, the present chapter holds that we are affected by the space and this is usually to the entire situation even in the pandemic period where people must have a new attitude that with time became incorporate in our sensorial modus.

And the effect to be 'affect by' is essential to understand the way we react to singular situations. It also allows proving that the relationship that we have with the surrounding environment is effectual in a typology of 'fleshly space' that in the logic of ambience theory we can perceive from the sensible point of view that unites us to the urbanity. The urban space isn't conceived as an anthropocentric dimension but, instead, through the re-valorization of daily life in congruence with the living space. We can also talk about the effect of topophilia that the geographer Yi-Fu Tuan (1974) illustrated as the perception of the environment that concerns the place with which the individuals have an affection relation and feel to be linked. To be attached is one of the keys to understanding the potentiality of the urbanity because the human being needs an intimate relationship with the city and environment that create, at the same time, the condition to be related with the others.

Also, within the effects of the pandemic situation, where many discourses are centred on a catastrophic point of view that announces (again) the 'death of the city' and social relation, the city endures being the sensible container of the lived experience of which the Being needs just to be in the world. The Being adapts itself to all kinds of situations and the street, the places, the spaces are a prothesis of ourselves; the condition of reality shows us that the sociality is the way to support the world. Then, sociality is the hope to redefine the construction of reality also with the consideration of the importance of digital dimensions. The interconnection with a new arrangement of the interior spaces that are more than more windows open on the world. In substance, the city must be perceived as a body. This requires a change of paradigm that finished with the obsessive vision of functionalist planning and achieve the perception of the organic city with all its pores that exude the vitality and made manifest the urban epidermis. 'This is the way, step inside'[2]....

---

[2] This is a verse of the song *Atrocity Exhibition* by Joy Division (1980).

REFERENCES

Bachelard G. (1957). *La poétique de l'espace*, Paris, PUF. Eng. Transl. by Maria Jolas, *the Poetic of Space* (1969). Boston, Beacon Press.

Benjamin, W. (1998). *Images de pensée* [*Images of the Thinking*]. Paris, Christian Bourgois.

Berque A. (2000). *Écoumène, introduction à l'étude des milieux humains* [*Ecumene, Introduction to the study of human environments*]. Paris, Belin.

De Certeau M. (1980). *L'invention du quotidien*. Paris, Gallimard. Eng trans. *The Practice of Everyday Life* (1984). Translated by Steven Rendall. Berkeley. University of California Press.

Di Felice M. (2010). *Paesaggi post urbani. La fine dell'esperienza urbana e le forme communicative dell'abitare* [*Post-Urban Landscapes. The end of the urban experience and the communicative forms of living*]. Milano, Bevivino.

Di Felice M., Cutolo Torres J., Yanaze L. (dir.) (2012), *Redes Digitais e Sustentabilidade. As interações com o meio ambiente na era da informação* [*Digital Networks and Sustainability. The Interactions with the Environment in the Information Age*]. São Paulo, Annablume.

Di Martino, E. (1977). *La fine del mondo. Contributo all'analisi delle apocalissi* [*The End of the World. Contribution to the analysis of apocalypses*]. A cura di Clara Gallini. Torino, Einaudi.

Fontana, A. (2020). *Ballando con l'apocalisse. I nuovi cittadini, i nuovi brand, i nuovi mondi nell'era dei cambiamenti catastrofici* [*Dancing with the apocalypse. New citizens, new brands, new models in the epoch of catastrophic changes*]. Macerata, Roi Edizioni.

Gibson, J.J. (1979). *The Ecological Approach to Visual Perception.* Boston, Hougton Mifflin.

Guattari F. (2013). *Qu'est-ce que l'écosophie?* [*What is the ecosophy?*]. Paris, Lignes.

Heidegger, M. (1927). *Sein und Zeit.* Eng. Transl. *Being and Time.* Translated by John Macquarrie, London, SCM Press, 1962.

La Rocca, F. (2013). *La ville dans tous ses états.* [*The city in all of its forms*]. Paris, CNRS Éditions.

Maffesoli, M. (1988). *Le temps des tribus.* Paris, Méridiens-Klincksieck. Eng. Transl. *The Time of the Tribes.* London, Sage, 1996.

Maffesoli M. (2017). *Ecosophie.* [*Ecosophy*]. Paris, Cerf.

Mauss, M. (1921). "L'expression obligatoire des sentiments (rituels oraux funéraires australiens)" [The compulsory expression of feelings (Australian funeral oral rituals]. *Journal de psychologie*, n°18, p. 425-434.

Moreno, C. (2020). *Droit de cité. De la "ville-monde" à la "ville du quart d'heure"* [*The Right of City. From the "world city" to the "city of the quarter of an hour*]. Paris, Édition de l'Observatoire.

Næss, A. (1989). *Ecology, community and lifestyle.* Cambridge, Cambridge University Press.

Næss, A. (2017). *Une écosophie pour la vie* [*An ecosophy for the life*]. Textes réunis par Hicham-Stéphane Afeissa. Paris, Seuil.

Rosa, H. (2019). *Resonance: A Sociology of Our Relationship to the World.* Cambridge, Polity Press.

Simmel, G. (1903). *Die Großstädte und das Geistesleben, Dresde, Petermann.* Trad. *The Metropolis and Mental Life.*

Tisseron, S. (2003). *L'intimité surexposée* [*The overexposed intimacy*] Paris, Ramsay.

Teyssot, G. (2009). *"Fenêtres et écrans: entre intimité et extimité"* ["*Windows and screen: between intimacy and extimity"*]. Revue Appareil. https://doi.org/10.4000/appareil.1005.

Tuan, Y. F. (1974). *Topophilia. A study of environmental perception, attitudes and values.* New Jersey, Englewood Cliffs, Prentice Hall.

In: Emotionality of COVID-19 ISBN: 978-1-53619-534-7
Editors: M. Korstanje and S. Adrian © 2021 Nova Science Publishers, Inc.

Chapter 7

PANDEMIC, SOCIAL POLICIES AND EMOTIONS IN THE METROPOLITAN AREA OF BUENOS AIRES

Angélica De Sena*
CONICET-UNLAM-UBA

... as is often the case, observing current events illustrates the understanding of the past and delving into what has happened clarifies what is happening: many of the Interdependence mechanisms of our days continue the changes of the past ... (Elias, 1993).

ABSTRACT

The Metropolitan Area of Buenos Aires is one of the poorest areas of Argentina. In this area is located La Matanza, the largest geographic municipality with the largest population and greatest vulnerability, as indicated by data from a pre-pandemic investigation. In March 2020, in Argentina the "social, preventive and mandatory isolation" was declared

* Corresponding Author's E-mail: angelicadesena@gmail.com.

in the face of the Covid-19 pandemic, which meant an increase in poverty and social assistance. In this context, an online survey study was carried out (in four waves: April, May, June and September/October) in order to ascertain the changes in the poverty situation of the population of La Matanza among the people receiving a social benefit, and related emotions around the pandemic and their own situation of vulnerability. For this, the exposition of the article will be: a) a review of the social and economic situation of the territory in question pre-pandemic; b) development of the theoretical perspective regarding social policies to address poverty in connection with emotions, considering social interventions that construct meanings, elaborate perceptions, and are located in the performativity of the aforementioned policies; c) development of the methodological aspects of research and analysis of quantitative information, taking into account the population that receives a social program and the emotions that emerge in relation to the pandemic. In this way, this chapter aims to make a substantial contribution to understanding the impact on the sensitivities of the recipients of the social interventions implemented in the context of a pandemic.

Keywords: pandemic, social politics, emotions, La Matanza, poverty

1. Review of the Pre-Pandemic Social Question in the Territory of La Matanza

Greater Buenos Aires is an area that surrounds the City of Buenos Aires, made up of 24 districts[1]; which as a whole form an "urban area," since they make up the largest urban complex in the country. According to the last census of 2010 (INDEC), the city concentrates almost 25% of the country's inhabitants. This region not only represents the largest single segment of the population, but is also where the highest levels of poverty and indigence are concentrated. In 2019, poverty affected 39.84% of the people who live in this area, and in the first quarter of 2020, with the start

[1] It is necessary to consider that the National Institute of Statistics and Censuses (INDEC) mentions 24 districts in the official website of the Autonomous City of Buenos Aires (https://www.buenosaires.gob.ar/gobierno/unidades%20de% 20projects% 20especiales% 20y% 20puerto / que-es-amba) are indicated 40 and, the CIPPEC 31. These distinctions run the limit towards municipalities traditionally considered of rural type, called "inland."

of quarantine due to the COVID-19 pandemic, it reached 47.5% (INDEC). The municipality of La Matanza, located in this region, is characterized not only by being the most populated - in 2010 it reached 1,772,130 people in a total of 483,397 homes (INDEC)- and extensive with 325.71 kilometers squares, but because it has a deep spatial segmentation that, in principle, can be subdivided into three large areas that are very different in terms of their socio-housing, economic and cultural characteristics. The first of these areas is that bordering the Autonomous City of Buenos Aires, where the inhabitants have more possibility of accessing drinking water and sewer services, it has most of the paved streets. The presence of villages and settlements is focused on relatively small sectors since they present to a lesser extent in comparison to the following areas. It is the area with the highest tax collection and the lowest rates of poverty and indigence due to the fact that it is the area that has achieved the greatest development over the years. The second zone has an intermediate population density. Only in recent years was the coverage of drinking water and sewers expanded, only half of the streets are paved and tax collection is irregular and/or poor. The third area is the one with the greatest vulnerability, where there are the greatest infrastructural and social deficits, the possibility of accessibility to services, educational and health centers decrease compared to the other areas, with the highest poverty index and the one furthest from the City Buenos Aires. Precarious employment and housing conditions deepened in the 1990s and have spread, with alterations, to date, generating new configurations in existing social networks. The district stands out for the development of grassroots organizations and social movements that emerge as a strategy to achieve occupation processes and popular settlements (Manzano, 2007; Barna, 2014).

In order to establish a map of the situation of social and economic vulnerability of the district, a description of the habitation conditions will be presented, considering the overcrowding conditions, access to services, working conditions and reception of social programs, ending with the elaboration of an index regarding the basic living conditions of the homes of La Matanza.

Following the results of our investigations[2] prior to the pandemic, we have identified that the district presents a deep segmentation and spatial segregation among the three aforementioned zones (PELM, 2005, De Sena et al. 2020). Regarding the issue of habitation, 122 informal settlements were identified (TECHO, 2016)[3], mostly in the second and third zones. It is in this sense that we have found that the population in the worst socio-economic situation, the one located in zones two and three, is the one that must buy water for cooking, and the one that has least access to sewers, with only 3.1% of homes in zone three having such access. In this framework, it is noted that 8% of the homes are in critical overcrowding conditions.[4]

La Matanza is a district of humid areas, bathed by a large number of streams and the Matanza-Riachuelo river. These streams and waterways cross large areas, which generate floods and contamination[5], so living nearby can mean damage to homes and human health. We have observed that in a third of La Matanza the neighborhoods have a stream nearby. This is more serious in the second and third zones where almost half of the neighborhoods have a nearby stream. In this sense, the news regarding floods are frequent. We have detected that 43.6% of the lands are flooded. This information is completed with two more elements: the existence of storm drains in the neighborhood and the type of streets (paved or dirt). The storm drains serve to collect the water derived from the rains and prevent floods from occurring. In this municipality, a third of the neighborhoods do not have storm drains, a situation that worsens in the second zone - 58.3% do not have it - and in the third, 57.1% do not have it. This set of factors begins to explain the floods, but the public health problems they cause also deserve attention (De Sena et al. 2020). Along

---

[2] We refer to the quantitative and qualitative project: "Main features of the" social question "at the beginning of the XXI century. La Matanza 2017-2019." (PROINCE) PIDC code 55 B 206. National University of La Matanza. 2017-2018; under the direction of Angélica De Sena. The data presented here respond to a household survey witnessed, with a probabilistic sample of 829 households throughout the municipality of La Matanza.

[3] http://relevamiento.techo.org.ar/index.html.

[4] Critical overcrowding: corresponds to households with more than three people per room. For the calculation here, three or more people were taken to determine overcrowding.

[5] http://www.acumar.gob.ar/caracteristicas-cuenca-matanza-riachuelo/.

with this, the industrial discharge without previous treatment, and the clandestine dumping of garbage, is not only a constant factor of contamination of the Matanza river, but also of the water courses of the tributary streams in the district, especially Arroyo Morales, the longest within the district's territory (PELM 2005).

Regarding the employment situation, it was identified that 52% of the working population does so in informal conditions and most of the occupations refer to semi-skilled and unskilled activities. It is possible to observe some differences by gender. For example, a third of women perform cleaning tasks, and 14.1% of men are street vendors or laborers. And the situation is always more unfavorable for the second and third zones (De Sena, 2019).

Regarding the means of income that the household has, we have observed that 16% lack a regular monthly income, and that they subsist on exceptional income or due to debt, evidencing the precarious situation in which life develops.

Regarding the socio-economic level[6], where ABC1 refers to the high level, with better economic and social position, the medium-high and medium-low level C2 and C3 respectively, and the low level divided into D and E refers to the low-high and low-low respectively. In La Matanza, the results indicate that 69.6% of the homes are of low socioeconomic level, and only 1.2% reach the high level and 23.7% the medium level. When reviewing the socio-economic level according to the area where the home is located, it is observed that the small percentage that achieves the ABC1 level is essentially located in the first area. While it is relevant to note that level E, in the first zone reaches 25.1%, in the second 39.4%, reaching 48.2% in the third. In other words, although the population in general is of a low socio-economic level (almost 70%), almost half belongs to the third zone.

---

[6] This was taken as a base model *NSE* simplified (Socio-economic Level) questionnaire, corresponding to the year 2015 (latest version), of the Argentine Society of Marketing and Opinion Researchers (SAIMO). For this, the following variables were considered: income (considering the values of the total basic basket according to INDEC); medical coverage; level of studies achieved; working condition; and type of work activity.

Finally, and with the aim of broadening the view, we elaborated an index that would allow us to determine living conditions in a multidimensional way. Understanding by "basic living conditions" of a person the ways in which they develop their individual and social existence, linked to economic, health, education, employment and habitat aspects. Based on this, the following dimensions were designed: a) employment, whose indicators refer to the condition of activity and quality of employment; b) economic sustainability, in this case the indicators are related to the origin of the household income (work, social programs) and the receipt of different products (food, medicines, etc.); c) access to health, which refers to having some type of medical coverage and accessibility as distance from the health center or hospital[7]; d) education, taking into account the educational level of the respondent and the schooling of boys and girls in the home; e) housing, the level of overcrowding and access to health services were considered as indicators; and f) the environment of the home, in this case the indicators are related to the neighborhood conditions (garbage collection, flooding streets, storm drains, and nearby public transportation, among others). Based on this, the results obtained indicate that only 58% of households have basic living conditions; of the remainder, 3.1% do not possess these, and 39% only partially have them. This situation worsens in the second and third zones, where only 47.8% and 44.1% respectively have basic living conditions.

It is in this context that we identify that in 26.2% of the households at least one person receives a social program to address poverty, and in these households the index showed lower results. Among households where there is a social program, only 22.9% have basic living conditions, while where there are none, almost 70% have such conditions.

The data presented so far show that the entire municipality of La Matanza prior to the Covid-19 pandemic was clearly exposed to deficient social and economic conditions. This situation is even more serious among people who receive a social program to address poverty[8] . In this context of

---

[7] This is a relevant indicator considering the geographical distances of the municipality and the inequalities between the first, second and third zones.

[8] 76% receive a cash transfer and they are women (Dettano, 2020).

high vulnerability, with a high percentage of people living from informal jobs[9] and with social programs, that is why we wonder about the impact of the Covid-19 quarantine and the emotions associated with it in this population.

Table 1. Basic living conditions according to whether or not they have received programs to alleviate poverty, from the Matanza district, in percentages

Basic living conditions	General population	Households with at least one person receiving a SP	Households without receiving a SP
Has	54.9%	22.9%	69.4%
Partially has	39%	65.6%	30.2%
Does not have	3.1%	11.5%	0.4%
Total	100 (829)	100 (216)	100 (613)

Source: Own elaboration.

In the next section, a review of the theoretical perspective regarding social policies to address poverty in connection with emotions will be carried out, considering social interventions that build meanings, elaborate perceptions, considering the performativity of the aforementioned policies.

2. Emotions, Social Policies and Poverty

The social question approached as an aporia between formal equality and inequality of the Modern State (Castel, 1997) or as the contradictions of the Welfare State in capitalism (Offe, 1990), is associated with the social policies as interventions from the State towards the population in

[9] The informal workers mentioned must be added to the recipients of social programs who, in order to improve their income (given that according to our inquiries the subsidy only occupies the place of a "help") perform roles such as domestic workers, street vendors or other unskilled activities (Dettano, 2020).

order to tend towards the *welfare* of the population and/or to suture market failures.

The question regarding what social policies are has been widely problematized from different disciplinary spaces - essentially the economic and social - and linked to the Welfare State, considering the strong presence of the State in people's daily lives since it is the one who assigns and redistributes the resources. Therefore, social policies will affect the production and reproduction of life and therefore in the construction of our daily lives, whether they aim to ensure certain minimum levels and certain opportunities to all members of the community (Hegenbuch, 1958, in Titmuss, 1981), or as an attempt to direct the life of society along a path that it would not follow if it were allowed to run its course (Lafitte 1962, in Titmuss, 1981), or as state actions that contribute to the reduction of social conflicts ensuring the temporary persistence of the capitalist accumulation regime (Fleury Teixeira, 1997; Faleiros, 2004; De Sena and Cena, 2014). In other words, beyond the definition of what we call social policies, these always refer to State interventions for specific purposes, which respond to the ideological conceptions of a given government, which intervene in the life of the community. Therefore, both the actions and the omissions of each social policy construct meanings and shape individual and social subjects, from which a social fabric is built and socialities are consolidated. In this way, if they are interventions that shape the conditions of production and reproduction of the life of the different sectors and social groups, then they condense the possibilities of naming meaning and doing (De Sena, 2016). We have already mentioned in other places that social policies have a normative character, that they also establish meanings, ways of seeing and feeling the world that perform the social question and structure emotions in the bodies of millions of subjects, as recipients, designers, and implementers of social policies (De Sena, 2016, De Sena and Scribano, 2020, Cena 2015, Dettano, 2017, Cena & Chahbenderian, 2012, Sordini, 2020, among others). For this reason, the sociological analysis of social policies from the perspective of bodies/emotions contributes to the study and understanding of the structuring mechanisms in contemporary capitalism. This is based on trying to combine a vision of these policies and how they build and consolidate ways of being, doing, thinking, and feeling, that structure the bodies and emotions in the subjects. There are intersections and articulations between the redefinitions of the "social question," the elaboration of social policies within the framework of the processes of state regulation of the conflicts between capital and labor, the necessary and desired sensitivities for this to happen, and the interventions of the agencies that are involved.

This means that social policies have a central place in defining the characteristics that the process of social production and reproduction will have in a given historical context, generating the conditions for it and for developing sociability. Therefore, these policies also operate in the symbolic aspects of life and in those associated with the cognitive-affective. In doing so, they institute and reproduce (causing, imposing, canceling and/or repressing) certain images, models and stereotypes of society, the subject, women, work, family, motherhood, among others, and emotions: anger, happiness, love, anger, fear. This configures the structure of sensitivities (De Sena, 2014, Scribano and De Sena, 2013) that affect the daily ways of living and the vicissitudes of the intervened subjects (Scribano, 2010).

The feelings and emotions experienced by the agents, as cognitive-affective practices, have an intertextuality linked to a specific historical and social context that corresponds to specific social situations (Luna Zamora, 2007, Scribano, 2007). "There is a necessary link between affective subjectivity and objective social situation" (Bericat Alastuey, 2000: 152) from where a set of emotions are induced in the actors, but also where controls that affect their feelings are incorporated. These norms are barely perceptible when *we feel what we should feel,* and we learn to manage the emotions corresponding to each moment, towards better social regulation (Scribano, 2007, 2012).

Therefore, the approach to the social question materialized in social policies It not only promotes or restricts certain emotions, but also the social implications of such affectation, that is, how to build the daily life from conditions of deficiencies, what will be the ideal "emotional competencies" to reverse them, to print them or to get used to them (Luna

Zamora, 2007; Hochschild 2011). Therefore, reviewing the emotions in the populations intervened through social programs leads us to understand the modes of social structuring. From these positions, in the following section, four surveys carried out during the quarantine by Covid-19 in the population receiving poverty care programs will be analyzed in order to uncover their emotions, as indicators that will allow us to later understand their practices.

3. Emotions, Social Programs, Quarantine and COVID-19

In this section we will analyze a series of results obtained from an investigation[10] that was carried out at the UNLaM in order to make visible some behaviors of the population of La Matanza against the restrictions established by the quarantine established in response to Covid-19. It was carried out through an online survey across four moments, the first from April 4 to 11, the second in May, the third in June, and the last at the end of September and the first days of October, from a non-probabilistic sample, based on a self-administered questionnaire with 3,291 respondents. The distribution ranged from the "snowball" technique to people over 18 years of age residing in the La Matanza district as part of the Greater Buenos Aires region. In this discussion, we will take as the focus of analysis the surveys completed by the people who receive a social program aimed at the alleviation of poverty (a total of 504 cases).

The year 2020 will be marked by Covid-19, with the first confirmed case in Argentina appearing on March 5, after which the number of infections increased rapidly, and on March 11 the World Health Organization declared the coronavirus outbreak to be a pandemic. In this context, and for the purpose of preventing the health system from collapse, on March 20 the Argentine national authorities established Social,

[10] Project "The social question in the party of La Matanza in the context of a pandemic." Vincular 2020 Program. UNLaM Rectoral Resolution No. 218/20. Secretariat of Science and Technology. National University of La Matanza. Director Angélica De Sena.

Preventive and Mandatory Isolation (ASPO) in decree 297/2020[11], known as "quarantine." The isolation was maintained -with some openings- until November 7, 2020,[12] the date on which the start of the stage of the "Social, Preventive and Obligatory Distancing" (DISPO) was announced[13] in the Autonomous City of Buenos Aires and Greater Buenos Aires Ulna (GBA), the area where the greatest number of cases and the longest period of isolation were concentrated. The ASPO decree limited the possibilities of mobility and travel along routes, roads and public spaces, and only tasks considered as *essential* could be carried out. So the cities were "closed," the streets were emptied, and we all had to "stay at home" in the face of ignorance of the behavior of the virus. One certain reality was the high level of contagion, and the only known means of prevention was a strategy of "isolation," a method that is not new and has been used in other pandemics over the years, such as the 'Spanish flu' of 1918.

This meant the closure of all face-to-face activities and only those related to food, hygiene and health were enabled. The rest compulsively entered virtuality. The advice that had to be followed were: "stay home," "wash your hands," "disinfect surfaces," and "keep distance between people." These councils were operationalized in a different way in the population, in relation to their social, labor, and accessibility conditions prior to the pandemic.

In the previous point we made mention of emotions as the result of the structuring and organization of life processes, tied to the different and multiple modes of State intervention, and particularly towards this population that receives interventions from a social program given their situation of poverty.

Elias (1993) refers to the relationship between the control of the subject in relation to emotional structures and how these are different according to social classes. Said control is made effective through the regulation of individual emotions by means of internal or external coercion and - in some way - the structures of human manifestations. In this way,

[11] See https://www.boletinoficial.gob.ar/detalleAviso/primera/227042/20200320.

[12] Therefore, the surveys were carried out in different months.

[13] According to Decree 875/2020, DECNU-2020-875-APN-PTE. Official Gazette https://www.boletinoficial.gob.ar/detalleAviso/primera/237062/20201107.

external coercion becomes internal and the different emotions (shame, fear, etc.) are structured as a certain continuous *self-control*, as unplanned configurations but in a specific order. Scribano (2009, Scribano and Vergara, 2009) refers to the mechanisms of social supportability and the devices for regulating sensations as a way of living life for those who are part of the world of No (no health, no education, no housing, etc.), but that in Argentina for some decades these have *not* been replaced with a massive array of social programs (De Sena, 2011).

Elías (1993) argued that emotions are made up of three major components, namely the somatic, behavior and feeling. For this reason, subjects faced with situations of uncertainty or danger prepare to face them by fighting or fleeing; it is in this sense that Scribano (2012) affirms that body/emotion are inseparable elements. In this way, it stresses those biologistic positions, constructionists or naturalists, with an approach that understands them as a result of social structuring processes. Hence, for Luna Zamora, emotions can be conceptualized as "learned schemes, reinterpreted, negotiated and functionalized or refunctionalized to structured and structuring sociocultural contexts (…) attention must be paid to the preconditions and structures that determine the experiences of certain emotions or other individuals who interact under these premises, defining and getting involved based on them" (Luna Zamora, 2005: 29). For this reason, although experienced individually, they are recognized by others in daily life and the State, based on the diverse and profuse modes of intervention, and this is constituted in the elaborator of a cognitive-affective text, in which social policies become the organizers of everyday life.

The ways in which modern states work, the configuration of societies, and the different institutions, all impact the moods of populations. The State configures a mode of sociability, which accentuates aspects such as joy, vivacity, happiness, cordiality, and kindness; inscribed in each historical context that grants a type of life experience, it elaborates a mode of interaction and exchanges (Simmel, 1939).

For this reason, we question ourselves about the behavior of the population that, as shown in point 1, find themselves in a situation of social vulnerability. The pre-pandemic economy was complex, with respect to the emotions associated with Covid-19.

In the pre-pandemic investigation, we investigated the people who receive a social program, and there are two indicators that we present here. The first question regards how it feels to receive a social program, and the highest percentage responses are: 22.6% that it is a "help"[14], 13.9% that it is a "relief," 8.7% "joy" and 7.8% "Anger, anger." In other words, in one way or another, the different ways of accounting for the emotions around the program refer to a further contribution to the family economy.[15] The next question refers to how they feel each day, to which the most frequent responses were: 20.7% mentioned feeling "joy," while 15.6% felt "sadness, pain or suffering." These are followed by 10.8% with "anger," 7.4% feel "good," 6.6% "tired" and 4.9% "happiness." In this way, we can observe that in everyday life in limited conditions, both contextual and individual, only a quarter (joy + happy) of the population mentions emotions related to well-being.

In this context, the quarantine restricts people's possibilities for carrying out their work activities, especially considering that they were informal, further limiting their meager income. This is so much so that 62.8% respond that their economic situation is worse after quarantine since their income is lower. This situation is more serious according to the area of residence. That is to say, although the situation is always bad - in line with what was mentioned in point 1- in the first zone for 56.5% their income decreased, in the second zone this was the case for 62.7%, and in the third for 69.2%. The economic situation worsened from the age of 40, among the ages of greatest work activity between 25 and 64 years, and among women. The income of this population was decreasing with the quarantine and associated with it the impossibility of carrying out the work activities in which they were previously engaged; but the high level of

[14] In this regard, see Scribano Adrian and Angélica De Sena (2018) "Aid as the central axis of policies for the sensitivity of conditional income transfers," in De Sena, A. (editor). *Social intervention at the beginning of the XXI century: conditional transfers in the global order.* ESEditor. Buenos Aires. Pp 253-284. Available in http://estudiosociologicos.org/portal/la-intervencion-social-en-el-inicio-del-siglo-xxi-transferencia-condicionadas-en-el-orden-global/.

[15] It is necessary to consider that most of the programs refer to a Cash transfer.

inflation in the Argentine economy must also be added.[16] It is in this context that it should be analyzed that only 37.5% of the population mentioned that "they do not leave their home," making it clear that the rest do, and possibly for some task related to improving their day-to-day life. This behavior was modified with the months of quarantine and the worsening of the economic situation for people who receive social programs.

	April	May	June	September	October
Your income is lower than before the quarantine	*52.4%*	*83.3%*	*72%*	*71.4%*	*73.3%*
Today your economic situation is worse than before the quarantine	*57.7%*	*58.3%*	*66.7%*	*67.1%*	*76.7%*

When asked why sustaining household expenses from quarantine only 5.9% can sustain all household expenses, while 54.5% can only sustain basic household expenses and 39.6% cannot even sustain expenses basic.

It is in this context that we will try to review the emotions of this population in relation to the first three months of quarantine (April, May and June) and then those of September/October, given that at that time, although the decree of isolation was still in force, according to our notes[17] field, the isolation was no longer fulfilled and the streets were already populated with people circulating.

We will first analyze the initial moment of the quarantine (surveys of April, May, June[18]). At this time, among the recipients of poverty care programs, the emotion that arises in the first months of quarantine is fear

[16] Inflation in Argentina is a long-standing problem, in 2019 it reached 53%. For 2020, inflation in April and May was 1.5% respectively, in June 2.2%, September 2.8%, and October 3.8%. The largest price increases are in food products (INDEC, 2020).

[17] Information emerged from the research team that resides in La Matanza.

[18] We refer to 329 cases.

with 48.8%, followed by anxiety with 26.5% and concern with a residual percentage of 1.2%[19].

But these emotions change as the days pass and the quarantine continues: fear decreases since the month of April when it reached 53.3%, and in the month of May it drops to 45.7%, and in June it falls further to 37.3%. Conversely with anxiety: in April it is 23.6%, in May it is 30% and in June it rises to 32.2%. A quick explanation is that people are getting used to living with the virus, but also have to carry the anxiety that living with it means.

In order to better understand these two emotions, we will review them with two indicators that bring us quite close to the living conditions of this population: one refers to the area of residence (first, second and third) and the other to the level of education achieved. Regarding the area of residence, in the first area (the most affluent) fear reaches 35.6%, in the second area 51.7% and in the third 53%, that is to say, when conditions are worse fear increases. Regarding anxiety in the first zone it reaches 35.6%, in the second to 20.2% and in the third to 25.9%; then this emotion is felt mostly in more favored socioeconomic areas.

Zone of residence	**First Zone**	**Second Zone**	**Third Zone**
Fear	35.6%	51.7%	53%
Anxiety	35.6%	20.2%	25.9%

Regarding the level of educational achievement in relation to fear of Covid-19: 57% had a low level of educational attainment[20], 43.1% had completed intermediary studies, and 35% had a high level of education. On the other hand, anxiety appears for 21.1% of those who had only reached a low level of education, it increases to 29.7% for those with intermediate levels of attainment, and 40% for those who have completed higher

[19] Although in this writing we refer only to the recipients of programs of attention to poverty in the face of Covid-19, we highlight that this relationship is inverse among non-recipients, with 35.5% feeling anxiety and 28.9% feeling fear.

[20] Low refers to those who reached primary schooling, medium those who managed to finish middle school, and high those with university studies.

education. In this way, it is observed that lower levels of formal education increase fear, and vice versa with respect to anxiety.

Studies achieved	Low	Medium	High
Fear	57%	43.1%	35%
Anxiety	21.1%	29.7%	40%

What has been said so far allows us to hypothesize that fear increases as living conditions are worse and anxiety is less.

To continue with our analysis, we will consider the emotions that arise in this population after completing the 6 months of isolation decreed by the national government. Although according to our studies of the population, compliance with isolation was in fact limited. In this period emotions not mentioned above arise. Thus, the emotions most mentioned in the face of Covid-19 by people[21] who receive a poverty care program are: fear amongst 25.1%, boredom amongst 18.3%, anxiety amongst 17.1% and worry amongst 15.4%. Concern previously was at only 1.25%, and with the continuity of the increase in cases and the permanence of the ASPO it increases. And, an emotion not mentioned above also appears such as boredom.

When analyzing according to the area of residence of the respondents, the same relationship is maintained as in previous months: in the first area, a lower percentage than in the third and the same as in the second. Concern tends to be less in more disadvantaged areas since in the first it reaches 20%, 11.5% in the second and 14.3% in the third.

	First Zone	Second Zone	Third Zone
Fear	23.1%	23%	30.6%
Boredom	15.4%	24.6%	14.3%
Anxiety	16.9%	16.4%	18.4%
Concern	20%	11.5%	14.3%

[21] In this case we refer to 175 cases.

Continuing with the same criteria, educational attainment was also considered. This indicator seems to have a behavior similar to that of previous months. Fear continues to be greater as the education achieved decreases (36.34% for low studies, 26.7% medium and 12.1% high). Anxiety is greater for those who have completed higher level studies (9.1% low studies, 16.7% medium, and 24.2% high). Concern also increased with education, reaching 21.2% in those with higher education and 13.6% for those with a low level of education. Meanwhile, boredom goes down with educational attainment, given that 27.3% of those reporting this emotion have low levels of education, 18.3% medium and 12.1% high.

Studies achieved	**Low**	**Medium**	**High**
Fear	36.4%	26.7%	12.1%
Boredom	27.3%	18.3%	12.1%
Anxiety	9.1%	16.7%	24.2%
Concern	13.6%	14.2%	21.2%

One more element to take into account is that 67% of the population who mention feeling afraid are aged between 25 and 44 years old. It is women (35.6%) who feel fear more than men (20.4%), while anxiety is almost the same between genders.

And finally, regarding the economic issue, among those who evaluate their economic situation worse than before the quarantine, 31.4% feel fear and 32.6% anxiety. Among the beneficiaries of programs who consider that their situation is better than before quarantine, 16.7% feel fear and 22.4% feel anxiety.

Economic situation	**Worse than before quarantine**	**Same as before quarantine**	**Better than before quarantine**
Fear	31.4%	34.9%	16.7%
Anxiety	32.6%	25.7%	22.4%

Fear is an emotion that has been identified prior to the appearance of Covid-19, in the narratives of this population associated with the social program as a triple structuring linked to chance, the government, and the instability of both access and continuity to these policies of attention to the situation of poverty (Cena, 2019).

Feeling fear constitutes an emotion intimately linked to everyday life. In terms of Koury's study (2017) of fears in the city, this emotion impacts the organization of daily life, directly or indirectly affecting the practices of populations. Complementarily, Luna Zamora (2005) maintains that fear is constituted in and from an emotional experience, the product of the interaction between individual agency, biology, biography and society.

Continuing with Elias (1993), violence and fear are two strong elements in the processes of historical changes and, as a counterpart, trust and tolerance, the latter two were not mentioned even once by the respondents. The quarantine established through a decree told us what it is allowed to do and what is not allowed, leaving room for the configuration of behaviors and their regulation; a new organization of fears.

> ... "the structure of fears is nothing more than a psychic response to the constraints that men exert on others within social interdependence. Fears constitute one of the ways of union -and the most important- through which the structure of society flows over individual psychic functions. The engine of this civilizational transformation of the behavior of the social constraints that operate on the individual, such as fears, is constituted by a complete modification of the social constraints that operate on the individual, by a specific change of the entire relational network, and above all, a change in the organization of violence" (Elias, 1993: 527-528).

The author refers to fear as a powerful element in the process of civilization towards the achievement of social prohibitions. These prohibitions rest on a "natural and historical" fear, but it is never natural but responds to history and the structure of social relations. Fear, then, serves as a mechanism of *social support* based on self-control and as a barrier to any conflict.

On the other hand, fear for some authors has a common thread with anxiety, although others try to separate it (Sierra, Ortega & Zubeidat,

2003). Anxiety appears linked to a forward action, this agitation or anxiety also leads to a state that does not allow calm. Anxiety appears on the one hand as an adaptive response, and on the other with a certain link to fear, although Marks (1986) differentiates it by linking it with some anticipation of future or unpredictable dangers, and as a consequence of capitalist structures of pessimism towards the future (Woods and Grant, 2006).

In this way we can continue to hypothesize that fear and anxiety are in relation to the material conditions of life, so that when these conditions are worse fear and anxiety are also. In other words, the strong interdependence between what Elias (1993) calls the "inner world" and the "outer world," forming interdependence networks, giving way to what the author calls the self-control apparatus.

According to Sauri (1984), fear is a ritual and symbolic process (not basic) whose purpose is to reduce anxiety in the facc of uncertainty, as regulatory mechanisms, in some cases it can be lurking until it leads to an extreme degree of terror or panic. When this happens, the subject abandons direct confrontation and starts to flee or becomes paralyzed (Saurí, 1984). Meanwhile, for Bauman (2008), "fear" deepens when it is dispersed, unclear and cannot be identified with a specific object or place and considers it responsible for the continuous state of fear of (liquid modernity). Finally, Geoffrey R. Skoll (2010) points out fear as functional to the interests of an elite that intends to extend its hegemony and for this, "global fear" is fundamental. From discourses of fear as a restrictive, but at the same time stimulating, political being, as a result of a capitalist state where many have little and most of the wealth produced is little distributed. In this state of constant conflict, fear works as a deterrent mechanism so that citizen demands are dispersed or at least cannot be organized as a coherent whole.

CONCLUSION

A few brief lines to reflect on Covid-19 and the modes of social regulation. The 21st century was embedded in a resounding way in our lives, illuminating to the point of being dazzling the precarious situations in which populations lived accustomed to lack. In this case in La Matanza as a sample of a Greater Buenos Aires, once a symbol of industrialization and now as a constant unease, vulnerabilities and precariousness: in education, in the type of work activity, socioeconomic level, access to housing, access to infrastructure and conditions of habitation (sewer, gas, storm drains, flood streets). This lack of access to services increases household living costs (purchase of water cans, gas from a carafe) and worsens sanitary conditions (floods, streams, lack of sewers). The situation of spatial segregation is combined with a certain favelization. And, poverty is presented as structural against which *the battle was lost*[22], where social programs "served as a cushion to moderate the increase in the number of poor"[23]

In this context, fear and anxiety, along with boredom and worry, constitute the threads that bind behaviors such as Weber's iron cage towards this population, where the quarantine in response to Covid-19 crystallizes the non-thematization of entering/leaving.

Fear conditions life, from here it is necessary to consider that it is the emotion most pronounced by the recipients of a social program, from the emergence of Covid-19 and the various modes of isolation in the global order. Fear as a coagulation mechanism of action (Scribano, 2007), in terms of Elias (1993) is established as a coercion that operates on individuals in the configuration of violence.

In this way, the 21st century, paraphrasing Elias in this "new civilization," opens the doors for a new emotional constraint, which encompasses the inner world; that is, not only the social construction of emotions but also the social construction of the world's perceptual apparatus, and with it the construction of sensation (Scribano, 2020).

---

[22] The Minister of Social Development of the Nation when announcing the increase in poverty due to the quarantine, indicated that "three generations of structural poverty, that is, intergenerational poverty in the same family" (https://dib.com. ar / 2020/09 / daniel-arroyo-it-is-evident-that-we-have-had-an-increase-in-poverty-in-pandemic /).

[23] Statements of the Minister of Social Development of the Nation, https: // www.lanacion. com.ar/economy/daniel-arroyo-poverty-nid2465769.

REFERENCES

Barna, A. (2014) "No hay como la palabra escrita para defender lo que uno hace: Usos de la producción documental en la gestión cotidiana de la niñez en el municipio de La Matanza" ["There is nothing like the written word to defend what one does: Uses of documentary production in the daily management of childhood in the municipality of La Matanza] *Intersecciones en Antropología*, vol. 15, núm. pp. 153-165. Tandil: Universidad Nacional del Centro de la Provincia de Buenos Aires Buenos Aires. Disponible en: http://www.redalyc.org/articulo.oa?id=179532230011.

Bauman, Z. (2008). *Miedo Líquido: la sociedad contemporánea y sus miedos líquidos.* [*Liquid Fear: contemporary society and its liquid fears*]. Buenos Aires: Paidos.

Bericat Alastuey, E. (2000) *"La sociología de la emoción y la emoción en la sociología"* (pp. 145-176). [*Sociology of Emotions and emotions on sociology*] Barcelona: *Papers* 62.

Castel, R. (1997) *La metamorfosis de la cuestión social.* [*The metamorphosis of the social question*] Buenos Aires: Paidos.

Cena, R. (2019) "Políticas sociales y emociones en el siglo XXI: reflexiones sobre el miedo en las poblaciones destinatarias de programas sociales." [Social policies and emotions in the 21st century: reflections on fear in target populations of social programs] in *Intersticios Revista Sociológica de Pensamiento Crítico*, v. 12 (2) 2019. (Pp 137-148). Madrid. Disponible en http://www.intersticios.es.

Cena, Rebeca (2015). "Políticas sociales, cuerpos y emociones a principios del siglo XIX en Argentina." [Social policies, bodies and emotions at the beginning of the 19th century in Argentina] in *Convergencia, 22*(69), 213-232. México: Universidad Autónomo del Estado de México.

Cena, R. y Chahbenderian F. (2012) "El crédito y el consumo como "condiciones" de contentar y contener a las poblaciones expulsadas." [Credit and consumption as "conditions" to satisfy and contain the expelled populations] in, *Boletín Onteiken,* (pp. 37 – 529). Noviembre de 2012. Córdoba: Estudios sobre Acción Colectiva y Conflicto Social. Disponible en: http://onteaiken.com.ar/ver/boletin14/1-4.pdf.

De Sena, A. (2011). "Promoción de Microemprendimientos y políticas sociales: ¿Universalidad, Focalización o Masividad?, una discusión no acabada." [Promotion of Micro-enterprises and Social Policies: Universality, Targeting or Massivity? not an argument finished] in *Revista Pensamento Plural., 4*(8), 36-66. Pelotas: Universidade Federal de Pelotas.

De Sena, A. (2016) "Políticas Sociales, emociones y cuerpos" [Social Policies, emotions and bodies]. in *RBSE – Revista Brasileira de Sociologia da Emoção*. v. 15, n. 44. (Pp. 173-185). Paraiba: GREM. Disponible en: http://www.cchla.ufpb.br/rbse/DeSenaDos.pdf.

De Sena A. & Scribano A. (2020) *Social Policies and Emotions. A Look from the Global South*. London: Palgrave Macmillan.

De Sena, A., et al. (2020) "Aproximaciones a la cuestión social en La Matanza: algunas dimensiones para su análisis." [Approaches to the social question in La Matanza: some dimensions for its analysis] *Colección Vincular CyT. VOL. 2,* Sociedad. La Matanza: Secretaria de Ciencia y Tecnología. Universidad Nacional de La Matanza. Disponible en: http://repositoriocyt.unlam.edu.ar/handle/123456789/462 http://repositoriocyt.unlam.edu.ar/handle/123456789/462.

De Sena, A (2019). Dossier Trabajo "Principales rasgos de la 'cuestión social' al comienzo del siglo XXI. La Matanza 2017-2018," [Main features of the 'social question' at the beginning of the 21st century. La Matanza 2017-2018] in *Boletín Síntesis Clave, número 144 Marzo 2019*. La Matanza: Observatorio Social. Universidad Nacional de La Matanza. Disponible en https://observatoriosocial.unlam.edu.ar/descargas/19_sintesis_144.pdf.

De Sena, A & Cena, R. (2014) "¿Qué son las políticas sociales? Esbozos de respuestas" (Pp. 99-126) [What are social policies? Response stubs]. in: De Sena A. (editora). *Las políticas hecha cuerpo y lo social devenido emoción: lecturas sociológicas de las políticas sociales.* Buenos Aires: Estudios Sociológicos Editora/Universitas. Editorial

Científica Universitaria. [*Politics made body and the social turned into emotion: sociological readings of social policies*.]

Dettano, A. (2020) "Las políticas sociales en el Municipio de la Matanza: una mirada de sus receptores," (pp. 139-160) [Social policies in the Municipality of La Matanza: a view of its recipients] in De Sena, Angélica, et al. (2020) "Aproximaciones a la cuestión social en La Matanza: algunas dimensiones para su análisis." *Colección Vincular CyT. VOL. 2*, Sociedad. La Matanza: Secretaria de Ciencia y Tecnología. Universidad Nacional de La Matanza. Disponible en: http://repositoriocyt.unlam.edu.ar/handle/123456789/462.

Dettano, A. (2017). "Prácticas de consumo y emociones de las destinatarias de programas de transferencias condicionadas de ingreso en la Ciudad de Buenos Aires" [Consumption practices and emotions of the recipients of conditional income transfer programs in the City of Buenos Aires], *Revista Novos Rumos Sociológicos*. Vol. 5, N° 8. (Pp. 8-32). Pelotas: Universidade Federal de Pelotas.

Elias, (1993) *El proceso de la civilización*. [*The process of civilization*] Buenos Aires: Fondo de Cultura Económica.

Faleiros, V. (2004) "Las funciones de la política social en el capitalismo" (pp. 43-70) [*The functions of social policies in capitalism*] in Borgianni, E. y Montaño, C. (compiladores). *La política Social Hoy*. Sao Paulo: Cortez Editora.

Fleury Teixeira, S. (1997) *Estado sin ciudadanos. Seguridad social en América Latina*. [*State without citizens. Social security in Latin America*] Buenos Aires: Lugar Editorial.

Hochschild A. (2011) *La mercantilización de la vida íntima. Apuntes de la casa y el trabajo*. [*The commodification of intimate life. Notes from home and work*] Buenos Aires: Ed. Katz.

Koury, M. (2017). "*Cultura Emotiva e Sentimentos de Medo na Cidade*." [*Emotional culture and feelings of fear in the city*] Documentos de Trabajo del CIES N° 8. JULIO – 2017. Buenos Aires: CIES Disponible en: http://estudiosociologicos.org/portal/wpcontent/uploads/2017/09/ Documento-de-Trabajo-8-JULIO-2017.pdf.

Luna Zamora, R. (2005). *Sociología del miedo. Un estudio sobre las ánimas, diablos y elementos naturales.* [*Sociology of fear. A study on the souls, devils and natural elements*] México: Universidad de Guadalajara.

Manzano, V. (2007) "De La Matanza Obrera a Capital Nacional del Piquete: Etnografía de procesos políticos y cotidianos en contextos de transformación social." [*From La Matanza worker to National Capital to Piquete: Ethnography of political and daily processes in contexts of social transformation*] Tesis Doctoral. Facultad de Filosofía y Letras, Universidad de Buenos Aires. Buenos Aires: MIMEO.

Marks, I. (1986). *Tratamiento de neurosis.* [*Neurosis treatment*] Barcelona: Martínez Roca.

Offe, C. (1990) *Contradicciones en el Estado de Bienestar* [*Contradictions of the Welfare State*] Madrid: Alianza.

PELM (2005) *"La Matanza identidad y futuro."* [*La Matanza identity and future*] Documento nº1 del Plan Estratégico de La Matanza. La Matanza: MIMEO.

Saurí, J. J. (1984). *Las fobias.* [*Phobias*] Buenos Aires: Nueva Visión.

Scribano A. (2007) *Vete tristeza... Viene con pereza y no me deja pensar!... Hacia una sociología del sentimiento de impotencia.* [*Go away sadness ... It comes lazily and does not let me think! ... Towards a sociology of the feeling of powerlessness*] Córdoba: CEA-UNC –CUSCH.

Scribano, A. (2009) "¿Por qué una mirada sociológica de los cuerpos y las emociones? A Modo de Epílogo." (Pp. 141-151) [Why a sociological look at bodies and emotions? By Way of an Epilogue]. In: Figari, C. & Scribnao, A. (Orgs.). *Cuerpo(s), subjetividad(es) y conflicto(s) Hacia una sociología de los cuerpos y las emociones desde Latinoamérica.* Buenos Aires: CLACSO-CICCUS. [*Body (s), subjectivity (s) and conflict (s) Towards a sociology of bodies and emotions from Latin America.*]

Scribano. A & Vergara G. (2009) "Feos, sucios y malos: la regulación de los cuerpos y las emociones en Norbert Elías" [Ugly, dirty and bad: the regulation of bodies and emotions in Norbert Elías], In *Caderno CRH,*

v. 22, n 56 (Pp 411-422). Maio /Ago 2009. Salvador: Universidade Federal da Bahia.

Scribano, A. (2012) "Sociología de los cuerpos/emociones" (Pp. 91-111) [Sociology of bodies / emotions] In *Revista Latinoamericana de Estudios sobre Cuerpos, Emociones y Sociedad.* N°10. Año 4. Diciembre 2012-marzo de 2013. Buenos Aires: CIES. www.relaces.com.ar. [*Latin American Journal of Studies on Bodies, Emotions and Society*]

Scribano, A (2020) *The colonies of the 21st century sensations, emotions and sensibilities*, in https://northernnotes.leeds.ac.uk/the-colonies-of-the-21st-century-sensations-emotions-and-sensibilities/.

Sierra, J.; Ortega, Virgilio; Zubeidat, Ihab (2003) "Ansiedad, angustia y estrés: tres conceptos a diferenciar" (Pp. 10 – 59) [Anxiety, anguish and stress: three concepts to differentiate] in *Revista Mal-estar E Subjetividade, vol. 3*, núm. 1, março, 2003. Fortaleza: Universidade de Fortaleza.

Simmel, J (1939) "El pobre" [The poor] in *Sociología. Estudios sobre las formas de socialización*. Buenos Aires: Espasa-Calpe Argentina S. A.

Skoll, G. (2010) *Social Theory of Fear: terror, torture, and Death in a Post Capitalist World*. New York: Palgrave Macmillan.

Sordini, V. (2020) "Sociabilidades y emociones en titulares de programas alimentarios" (pp. 23-43) [Sociabilities and emotions in holders of food programs], in Dettano, A (comp) *Políticas Sociales y Emociones: (Per) vivencias en torno a las intervenciones estatales.* Buenos Aires: Estudios Sociológicos Editora. Disponible en http://estudio sociologicos.org/portal/eseditora/. [*Social Policies and Emotions: (Per) experiences around state interventions.*]

Woods, A & Grant, T (2006) *Razón y revolución filosofía marxista y ciencia moderna Centro de estudios socialistas.* [*Reason and Revolution Marxist Philosophy and Modern Science Center for Socialist Studies.*] Buenos Aires: Colihue.

In: Emotionality of COVID-19 ISBN: 978-1-53619-534-7
Editors: M. Korstanje and S. Adrian © 2021 Nova Science Publishers, Inc.

Chapter 8

SENSIBILITIES OF EATING INSIDE: EMOTIONS AND FOOD PRACTICES IN A TIME OF A PANDEMIC

Aldana Boragnio[*]
Center for Research on Consumption,
Sensitivities and Creativity (CICSEC),
University of Palermo, Argentina

ABSTRACT

In the pandemic situation, where social distancing and confinement were presented as the main tools for its prevention, eating became confined to the inside of the home. For those who have a home to stay in, eating has been reinstated as a practice in the private sphere and as a need to be met while remaining indoors. Eating is a daily practice that produces and reproduces the body, and it is shaped from habits, norms and customs that are expressed in social sensibilities. At the same time, it is directly linked to the configuration of emotions as the body/food/hunger/emotions relationship unfolds in an unbreakable

[*] Corresponding Author's E-mail: boragnio@gmail.com.

continuum. While the diet is configured as a set of practices that are practices of the politics of sensibilities, food and commensality practices imply and express sociabilities and experiences. In this case, by knowing about diet, food practices and commensality, we will know how people put into practice specific knowledge about food to organize and regulate the planning, preparation and consumption of their daily meals in the context of isolation and of a new organization of time. Thus, knowing about diet and its practices will allow us to know the sensibilities and experiences in the context of a pandemic, where food practices take on a greater importance, since it highlights not only the possibilities of access, variation, diversification and consumption, but specific sensibilities around cooking, eating and the home. The objective of this chapter is to expose the sensibilities of eating in a time of pandemic in Argentina and Spain, based on a comparative study between the two countries. To do this, we conducted an online survey, self-administered during the first five weeks of isolation and confinement, and in-depth interviews with young people from the tenth week, seeking to discover the eating practices of isolation in articulation with the time/space relationship, which are configured from a politics of sensibilities as cognitive-affective practices of feeling in the pandemic world.

INTRODUCTION

The COVID-19 pandemic came as a surprise to many and was suddenly imposed, shifting from the news to mandatory confinement and isolation measures that not only immediately and strongly impacted the productive structure, but also immediately modified daily life in a way not previously known to many.

In Spain, the period of physical confinement and total social isolation due to COVID-19 –called the State of Alarm and Confinement (EAC, for its acronym in Spanish)– was established by Royal Decree 463/2020 on March 14, 2020, A few days later, on March 20, 2020, in Argentina, the Social, Preventive and Mandatory Isolation (ASPO, for its acronym in Spanish) came into effect. This new reality forced the subjects to not only modify their daily life, but also involved returning the home to the centre of all activities. Work, education, entertainment, training, and consumption were modified to be held indoors and in several cases, transformed to be able to be realized.

From the confinement and isolation policies due to the COVID-19 pandemic, food took on a new centrality in this context. First, it exposed the possibility of the lack of food amongst people who were born in the era of overabundance, while the fragility of the food system was exposed, reconfiguring this as an essential activity. During this period, eating was again configured as a practice inside the home, where, in many cases, it brought the subjects together again socially in the shared act. Thus, the reinstatement of eating as a practice in the private sphere and as a need to be answered on a daily basis within the home led to a readjustment of food practices and commensality.

The objective of this chapter is to expose the sensibilites of eating in a time of pandemic in Argentina and Spain, seeking to uncover the food practices and commensality practices in conjunction with the temporal/spatial relationship of confinement, which is configured from a policy of sensibilities as cognitive-affective practices of sentiment in the world of the pandemic.

The data presented comes from an online survey, self-administered, in which the food practices related to the purchase, cooking and consumption of food in households were investigated. The survey was carried out during the first five weeks after the implementation of the ASPO in Argentina and the EAC in Spain, obtaining 472 responses for the case of Argentina and 290 for Spain.

Secondly, from the tenth week of ASPO and EAC, in-depth interviews were conducted with young people from Spain and Argentina between 20 and 29 years old, since this age group was the one that offered the most responses to the survey. The main objective of the interviews was to collect information on the eating practices in isolation in conjunction with the temporal and spatial relationship of the period of exit from the prohibitions. Informed consent was requested to carry out the interviews and the anonymity of the participants was preserved. These were recorded and fully transcribed to be subjected to data analysis, classifying their content defined according to emerging themes.

The argumentative strategy will be as follows: a) a brief overview is offered of the relationship between body/emotions/eating from the standpoint of a sociology of bodies/emotions; b) the specificities of the concepts of food practices and commensality are explicated; c) the data from the surveys and interviews are presented, detailing the emotions around eating and the changes produced by confinement; and d) some final lines are presented by way of conclusion and identifying future openings for inquiry.

EATING BODIES/EMOTIONS

When we talk about bodies and food we talk about bodies that eat. We refer to biological bodies that need to ingest food and nutrients for their reproduction, but also to the emotions that are configured from the availability and appropriation of daily energies. This occurs without ceasing to relate the social relationships necessary for this to happen. Thus, eating is not only central to the reproduction and social availability of bodies, but the organic/cognitive/affective is intertwined in the production and reproduction of bodies/emotions.[1]

From the sociology of bodies/emotions, we understand that

> "The bodies are such, given their connection with the environment/environment (material conditions of existence) through (and by) the complex processes that are generated in the interaction between (with and from) the brain/central nervous system/nutrients/energies. b) The brain "houses" (in a complex and indeterminate way) the processes of the social construction of bodies and emotions mediated by a set of interactive modularities between the chemical and electrical "causes" of the life systems that articulate the capacities that have nutrients/energies to enable/block, produce/reproduce and/or balance/unbalance the existence of those bodies/emotions. c) The unequal distribution and appropriation of nutrients/energies model the potentialities that the

[1] The bar (/) implies the possibility of writing and inscribing the connections/disconnections that involve bodies and emotions and allows us to grasp/understand that seeing, tasting, smelling, hearing, feeling, perceiving, thinking, wanting, acting are complex, indeterminate moments and nodes through which the multiple subject/society relationships are woven (Scribano, 2012).

neurophysiological system has to "maintain" the possible states of life of the subjects as social agents. d) The processes of social structuring by "modelling" the possible connections between impressions/ perceptions/ sensations/emotions and the brain/energies/environment are variables that co-embody the possible forms of bodies/emotions" (Scribano 2012: 97).

From this conceptualization, it is possible to observe the limits of a society that becomes a body, while bodies will be produced and reproduced within the limits of the material conditions of existence that society distributes unequally among subjects. In this sense, the relationship between bodies/environment/nutrients is essential for the conformation of bodies, at the same time that it will enhance/block the perceptual, emotional and cognitive capacities of those bodies as they grow.

Emotions will allow the subject to feel (himself), which gives him the capacity for action, understanding it as "action tendencies instead of specific actions" (Von Scheve & Slaby 2019: 10). But, emotions are not the result of a single cause/motivation but rather "are the result of the co-bordering[2] of a constellation of previous interactions between multiple factors" (Scribano 2018: 7) and, in their indeterminacy and complexity, they emerge from the processes of adjudication and correspondence between perception/sensation/emotion.

At this point it is important to note that the sensations are distributed according to the specific forms of bodily capital that are the conditions of existence housed in the body, understanding it from three registers: a) an individual body, which refers to the body as a biological organism, as an organism that has organs, functions and processes that are genetically constituted; b) a subjective body, which is found in the field of the "I" that constructs a narrative of its existence as a biography - in this plane, interactions and relationships with others take place; and c) the social

---

[2] "Cobordism is basically an equivalence relation between compact varieties. Two varieties are said to be cobordant if their alien union is the border of a third compact variety. As we will see, the border of a variety of dimension n + 1 is a variety of dimension n, and the border of a variety with the border is a variety without border" (Pérez and Ávila, 2011: 3). The main problem with cobordism is "knowing when two varieties can be deformed into each other without encountering a singularity in the resulting space, at any moment in this deformation" (Thom, in Wiley & Sons Aubin 2004: 103).

body, which is the incorporation of learning, practices and habits that shape the body and that constitutes subjectivity from socialization (Scribano 2007).

This way of understanding the body with analytical distinctions that occur in an inter-crossed and superimposed way makes it possible to think of the connections between sensations and the body as a given state of affairs. In this way, the subject and her material conditions of existence are interconnected in dialectical tension with the result of feeling-in-a-body. For its part, talking about bodies implies talking about a politics of bodies, understood as "the strategies that a society accepts to respond to the social availability of individuals" (Scribano 2015: 35). In this case, the politics of bodies will organize socially accepted practices and strategies to respond to the daily need to eat in their relationship between bodies/environment/ nutrients.

On the other hand, all politics of the bodies implies a politics of sensibilities, which regulates how the actors experience the states of feeling and feeling the world. In this sense, the politics of sensibilities is linked to a

> set of cognitive-affective social practices aimed at the production, management and reproduction of horizons of action, disposition and cognition. These horizons refer: 1) to the organization of daily life (day-to-day, wakefulness/sleep, food/withdrawal, etc.); 2) to information used to order preferences and values (adequate/inappropriate, acceptable/ unacceptable, bearable/unbearable) and 3) to the parameters for time/ space management (displacement/location, walls/bridges; infrastructure for the valorization of enjoyment) (Scribano 2018: 10).

This interconnection allows us to understand that the body/food/ emotions relationship is a central node in the structuring of sensibilities since eating elaborates, inscribes and reproduces the possibilities of living and narrating the world based on the potentialities and obturation that are nested in the distribution of nutrients and energies, constituting the possibilities of feeling-in-the-world from a-body.

Eating Practices: Food Practices, Commensality and Sensibilities

Now, if we talk about eating, we refer to a practice that subjects carry out throughout their lives and that, under ideal conditions, they should repeat a couple of times a day. At the same time, it must be taken into account that this practice can be carried out from a complex system of relationships that ranges from the production of food to the intake itself.

Eating practices encompass elements of a cultural, economic, social and individual nature, which intersect with the actions necessary to reach the act of eating. On the one hand, we find food practices, which as "the actions of obtaining, accumulating, preparing, conserving food, together with the knowledge in this regard, held by a specific group in a specific historical context" (Boragnio and Sordini 2019: 74). And, on the other, commensality, which is organized based on habits, norms and customs.

Commensality is the way of eating typical of human beings. From omnivorism, and with the difficulties involved in obtaining the necessary food in solitude, sharing food became essential for the reproduction of the species, generating specific norms that constituted the moment of eating at the same time as a community of diners (Fernández-Armesto 2009; García 2013). Therefore, 'eating' is organized by cultural guidelines before the specific moment in which the food will be eaten. These guidelines will vary in each culture and will be modified according to gender, age, the social position of who eats along with the specific context of space/time where the act of eating will take place.

If commensality is the form acquired by sharing food among human beings, and if these forms are constituted by the set of social relations, the rules of commensality will focus on legitimate ways to carry out sharing. Thus, commensality has four main axes: rules/norms, time, space, types of interaction, the latter being the various ways of carrying out the rules/norms —every day, extra-daily, festive, in physical presence, alone—.

In western societies, from the twentieth century, the process of change called "food modernity" or "late modernity" began, in which commensality enters into crisis and the shared rules fall, producing a destructuring of eating behaviors (Fischler 1995, 2010; Contreras Hernández 2005). The entry of women into the labour market, the extension of school hours and working distances, the development of the food industry on a massive scale and the production of ultra-processed products, as well as the creation of a market segmented by income, they modified daily life, which led to changes in food practices.

The first modifications that were made focus on "de-structuring, de-socialization, de-implantation of hours and de-ritualization" (Poulain 2002). These "de-" tendencies are observed in three concrete practices of daily life: a) the simplification of the structure of food, making the dishes increasingly simple; b) the increase in consumption outside the home, making public a daily practice linked to the private; and, c) the increase in the number of ingestions, which separate the act of eating from a specific time, which amplifies both the hourly and spatial possibilities.

Within the framework of these changes, daily food tends to be linked to an extra load to the working day, which is quickly solved in the domestic environment, with ultra-processed industrial products. In this sense, food is no longer organized by family life, but rather, the strategies to provide a solution to the daily diet focus on individualism and the destructuring of intakes. In this way, "snacking"[3] appears as the form that the subjects give to the current diet (Mintz 1996; Poulain 2002).

Although current commensality is not strictly unstructured and guided by "snacking", the modernization of daily life, the value of time and the objectification of the body, have been continuously and deeply transforming the ways of eating, thinking and sharing the food. Thus, among the main changes in the rules of commensality is the shift of the choice of food to the individual scope, the loss of regulated times of eating, the increase in the number of times and the amount of intake, the

[3] Small portions of food or meals that are eaten at varied times, between main meals, but are not considered as a proper meal. Nutritionally the concept of snack is about what is called "junk food".

monotony of food, the loss of culinary know-how and the ritualization of food as a consumer experience (Boragnio 2020; Aguirre et al. 2015).

The richness of commensality as a concept does not reside only in the specificity of the act of sharing food and the rules that are involved in that act, but also in the plurality of meanings and modes that it possesses. So, as we can see, the experience of eating will be traversed by the politics of bodies and commensality. In this way, from before birth and reinforcing themselves in the daily act of eating, people are articulated with the social structure based on habits, norms and customs that are expressed in social sensibilities.

As we can see, eating practices have a dynamic character, so they are able to readjust depending on the context, but always within the sociocultural system that gives meaning to commensality. Next, we present the main characteristics of eating in Argentine homes, then the details and pictures of eating in Spanish homes will be outlined, and then we will focus on sharing the emotions and sensibilities linked to both countries.

EMOTIONS OF EATING AT HOME

Eating in Argentine Homes

When asking respondents what place food occupies in their lives, 76.4% of Argentines gave scores of 7 upwards, the mode is 8.

For young people from 19 to 29 years old, the mode about the level of importance of food is also 8, but the responses that indicated a value of 7 or more are 86%.

When the respondents were asked to indicate with three words what they felt when eating, the predominant responses, in order of frequency, were: satisfaction, good, happiness, tranquility, glad, very good, grateful, guilty, pleasure and normal. If we add the answers obtained for "good" and "very good" we can produce a category of "well-being" that would have the first place.

For their part, respondents aged 19 to 29 indicated that their feelings were mainly focused on satisfaction, happiness, good and glad. But we also find repeated responses such as enjoyment, calm, full, anxiety, energetic and healthy.

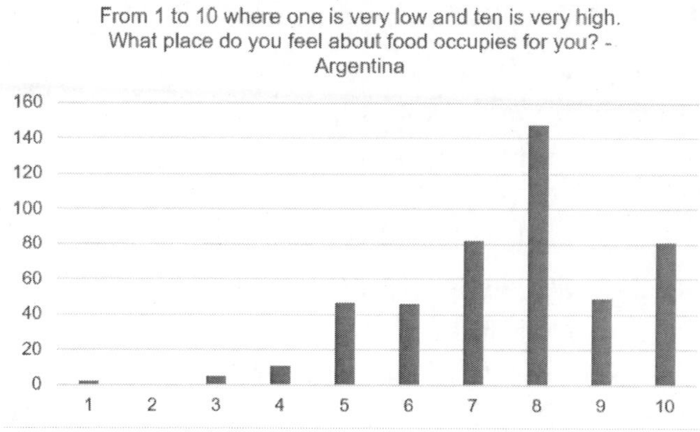

Figure 1. Place of food in life, Argentina.

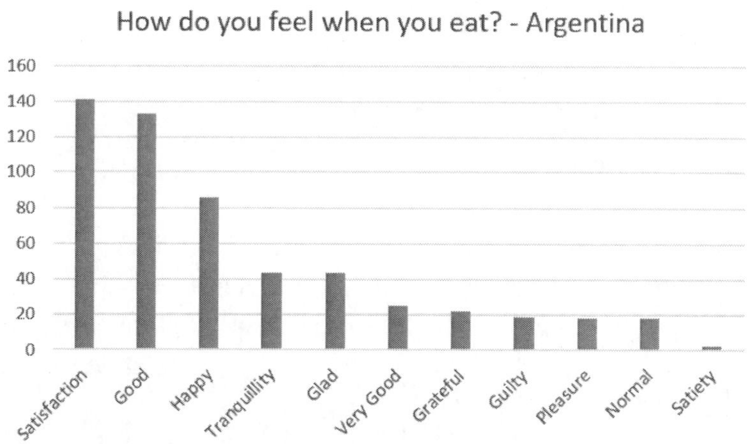

Figure 2. Emotions when eating in Argentina.

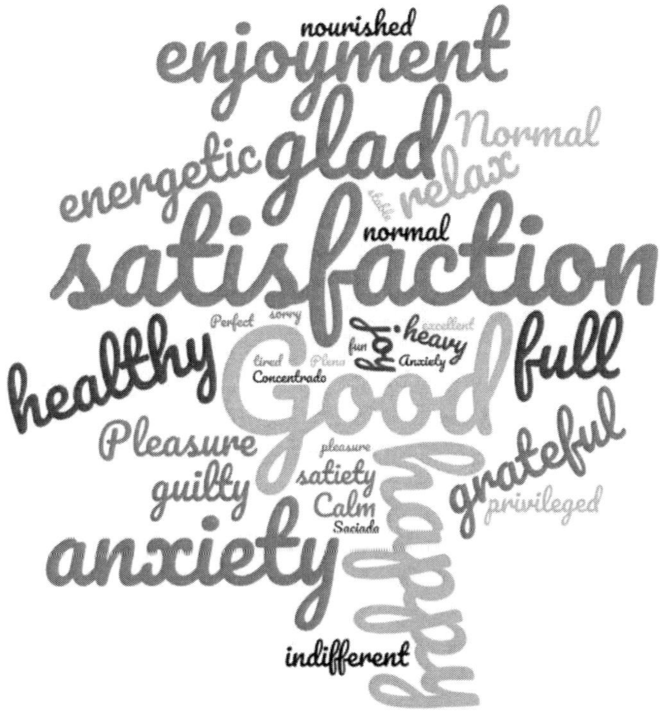

Figure 3. Word cloud of the responses of young people aged 19 to 29 in Argentina.

Eating in Spanish Homes

When asking Spaniards what place food occupies in their lives, 84.55% gave scores higher than 8, this being the mode.

For young people from 19 to 29 years old, the mode with the level of importance of food is also 8, but the responses that indicated a value of 8 or more are 63%.

When the Spaniards were asked what they felt when they ate, the predominant responses, in order of frequency, were: good, satisfaction, happiness, glad, satiety, gratitude, full, at ease, relaxed, calm. Feeling 'good' ranks first, almost sharing frequency with satisfaction and happiness.

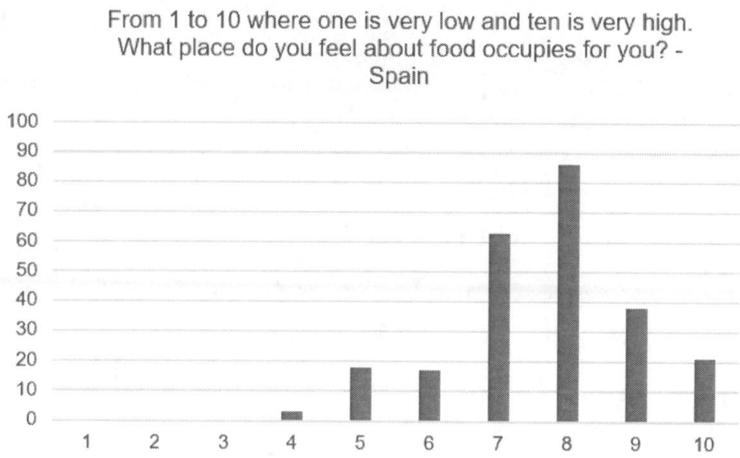

Figure 4. Place of food in life, Spain.

For their part, respondents from 19 to 29 years old indicated that their feelings were mainly focused on good, happiness, satisfaction, comfortable and glad. But we also found several important responses in full, anxiety, guilty, grateful, satiety, guilty and enjoyment.

Focusing on the comparison between countries, we see that, when asked about the place of importance of food, in both countries, the number was 8 with 31.35% for Argentina and 36% for Spain.

About the emotions related to eating of all the survey participants, we can observe that, in both countries, the three most repeated emotions are: well-being, satisfaction and happiness.

On the other hand, in a population of 19 to 29 years of age in both countries, responses are the same. In Argentina, the three most repeated emotions are satisfaction, good and happy, while in Spain they are also good, happy and satisfaction. As for differences, we find that young people from Argentina also indicate feeling glad, enjoyment, anxiety, full, healthy and grateful; while young Spanish people feel comfortable, grateful, satiety, full, guilty and healthy.

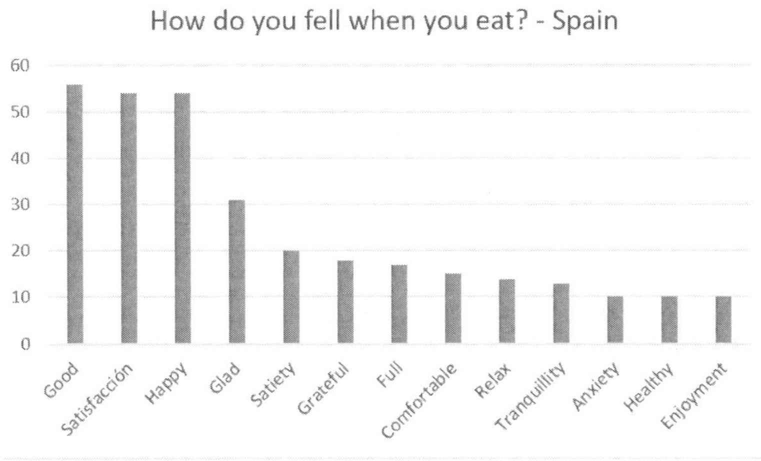

Figure 5. Emotions when eating in Spain.

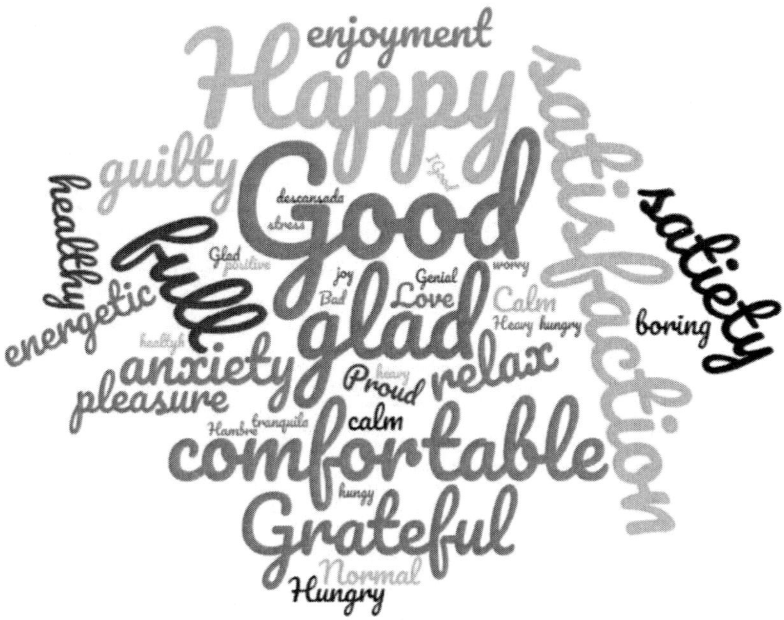

Figure 6. Word cloud of the responses of young people aged 19 to 29 in Spain.

EATING IN TIMES OF CONFINEMENT

When analyzing the data from the surveys and interviews together, new axes appear to take into account when thinking about the eating practices at home in times of pandemic. Among the main changes shown by the data are not only changes in what is eaten, but also in food and commensality practices.

The first modification that appears as a positive change and, at the same time, as a negative change for the research participants, is the routine of schedules. The changes in the schedules are expressed mainly in the fact of skipping a meal as in the incorporation of breakfast daily.

> "I consume less purchased food, more snacks and breakfasts, also simpler meals" (26-year-old female, Argentina)
>
> "I have disorganized schedules, I eat junk food in excess as a snack" (29-year-old female, Spain)

Thus, the change in schedules allowed the subjects to organize the day, but as we can see, it also disorganized it.

On the other hand, schedule changes are directly related to changes in the menu. First appears the need to plan different menus since having to eat every day at home, taking charge of the entire purchase/planning/cooking process, and the need to innovate are imposed so as not to fall into monotony. As the interviewees tell us:

> "I cook more, I got out of the dynamic of always eating the same thing." (28-year-old female, Argentina)
>
> "I believe that at some point during this quarantine we have all made, even if it is an attempt to cook, that, although you are not always cooking throughout these days, you have tried. (…) The week has 7 days, you have to be cooking the same thing so to speak, but in 7 different versions." (25-year-old female, Spain)

These variations in the dishes were not only introduced by the need to eat other things, but could be achieved by the time available, which offered the possibility of cooking new things, of being able to dedicate time to the kitchen and more complex preparations.

> "I like to vary from what I always eat because I have more time to look at recipes and cook them." (23-year-old female, Argentina)
>
> "Take advantage of the time to make healthier and more elaborate meals." (24 -year-old female, Spain)

Based on this, surveys show that the new preparations made in Argentina and Spain focus on the mains, sweets, followed by dishes that were frequently consumed, but made in a homemade way. With this, the interviewees indicate that they began to cook as a new quarantine practice, and those who already cooked before took advantage of the time to make more elaborate and complex dishes.

> "Instead of buying, it was replaced by making it at home." (24 -year-old female, Argentina)

In this case, it is striking that in surveys in Spain pride appears as an emotion linked to eating in a pandemic, since respondents were able to realize that they can cook and do it well.

> "I am proud of the menus that I am making, but stressed by the amount of flour." (21-year-old female, Spain)

Along with the kitchen, there is the stress of flour consumption and the multiple strategies to limit its consumption and implement and sustain the consumption of healthy foods. About this, in the surveys, it can be observed that the search for a healthy diet is one of the main axes, either to stay healthy at this stage, to avoid getting sick, and not to gain weight. For this, respondents and interviewees tell us they choose light, healthy foods.

> "I vary foods to maintain a balanced diet weekly." (20-year-old female, Argentina)

> "I try to maintain a balanced diet (salad, baked vegetables)." (24-year-old female, Spain)

At the same time, although most of the answers about the diet in the days of isolation focused on being happy and satisfied with it, it was also clearly emphasized that there was something wrong and it was marked as something to be modified.

> "Although I did eat and we eat super healthy, I know that we ate unnecessary sweet things." (23-year-old female, Argentine)
>
> "Are you satisfied with your diet these days?
>
> No, I would like to eat healthier." (23-year-old female, Spain)

In this sense, several respondents said they were on a diet and/or going to a nutritionist. Among those who said they consulted a nutritionist, almost all went before the isolation period and tried to maintain the diet.

> "It depends on what you are eating. When I eat every day I feel good, and I like to eat balanced and think about combining different foods. When I eat something out of the ordinary (something more "fattening") I enjoy it a lot at the moment and eat everything I think I want but knowing that later I will be blamed or I will feel very full." (woman, 24 years old, Argentina)
>
> "It depends on what you eat. If I eat healthily I feel good. If I go off my diet I feel guilty, bad." (28-year-old female, Spain)

We understand the need to go to the doctor to learn how to eat as the loss of knowledge concerning eating practices occurs from multiple factors within food modernity. On the one hand, due to the separation between the social norms of eating, the separation of food production, the reorganization of the times where it is no longer clear what is eaten at what time and the deregulation that occurs from individualism to eat alone. Then, the cacophony (Fischler 1995) generates an excess of discourses that have as consequences the uncertainty about which one to follow, since all are expressed under the label of "the truth". This, added to the medicalization of food that led to the de-hierarchization of women in eating issues (Boragnio 2020b), which place them as the unauthorized voices and, therefore, in the space of non-knowledge. But, at the same time, we observe that this time of change in the period of the ASPO and the EAC, provided the possibility for the youngest to approach the kitchen as a way of doing, of transforming daily life, not only not to be "eating the same" but to try to "feel good."

BY WAY OF CONCLUSION: SENSIBILITIES OF EATING INSIDE

The confinement and isolation decreed by the spread of COVID-19 led to a rethinking of food practices and commensality, configuring eating practices as a central node of daily life during the pandemic. In this case, eating as a daily act that had been turned into the public sphere –from the implementation of multiple modifications in domestic, school and work-life– was redirected to the interior of the home, once again becoming a domestic and family activity. From this change, new rules of commensality were generated. On the one hand, this centered around the types of interaction that became entirely domestic and every day. And, on the other, they were configured in relation to the time and space that allowed subjects, in some cases, to re-order the daily diet.

The period of confinement and isolation brought young people closer to the practice of cooking, generating emotions of satisfaction and pride. As the body/food/emotion relationship develops, we can observe that the action of cooking seeks well-being, satisfaction and containment. But at the same time, the introduction of the multiple discourses, of a politics of sensibilities around "nutrition", reproduces the idea of not knowing how to eat. At the same time, the practice of eating is configured as an individual learning activity. In this way, the experience of eating is articulated in young people between guilt, anxiety and enjoyment.

Nutritional sensibilities organize and classify preferences and values where health is put first when choosing what to eat. Eating is no longer organized based on calendar dates or family knowledge, but eating practices are structured by a mediated medicalization based on nutritionism configured as a sensibility to eating. Thus, the diet is configured as a set of practices that are practices of the politics of sensibilities, while the food practices and commensality imply and express different sociabilities and experiences.

From the emotions linked to eating, we can observe the connection of this as a cognitive-affective social practice, which not only tends to the production and reproduction of the body in its materiality, but also to the production and reproduction of the individual and social energies that will constitute the possible horizons of action, disposition and cognition. Eating organizes daily life. In isolation, the day is spent thinking about what to eat, when to eat, what to do to eat. But, at the same time, eating orders the day, orders the hours, what is eaten during the day, at night, based on the rules and norms of commensality.

Finally, it is important to point out that, as we can see, eating is organized based on parameters for other time/space management. In this sense, in the period of isolation and confinement, when public time/space was unable to inhabit for many –while many others inhabited it without the possibility of autonomy or decision– domestic time/space was reconfigured and multiplied. At this time, cooking was once again the main axis of daily life at home. And although industrialized foods, service foods and ultra-processed foods continue to be the edibles that reproduce eating at home, the new time allowed other possible ways of eating to be explored. Whether they are reproducing what was consumed outside at other times or producing something new, the traditional, the common shared at home, the commensality that builds edibles into food.

In this way, from the eating conditions of life and its reproduction are molded –as nutrients configure the bodies and emotions– at the same time that the ways of experiencing eating and experiencing the body are defined by possible foods and their taste, diners are configured and social relationships are hatched. In this sense, the consequences of eating become evident in the structuring of sensibilities, based on regimes that constitute particular ways of regulating, ordering and incorporating social practices in specific socio-historical contexts.

Eating is a key determinant of people's health, but also of their daily emotional experience. This pandemic reality not only affects food practices and commensality, but also affects and configures the emotions. A long way ahead is the analysis of the eating practices of young people, to learn more about the diet that they put into practice, their knowledge and specific strategies for planning, preparing and consuming their daily meals, to know the relationships between body/food/emotions in the post-pandemic 21st century; with the final interest of being able to approach the transformations of the set of cognitive-affective social practices aimed at the production, management and reproduction of horizons of action, disposition and cognition. In other words, being able to know the policies of the sensibilities that are currently being formed.

The lines of inquiry presented in these pages allow us to continue deepening the interconnection in the relationship between body/food/emotions as the central node in the structuring of sensibilities, since eating elaborates, inscribes and reproduces the possibilities of living and narrating the world from the potentialities and obturation that are nested in the distribution of nutrients and energies, by constituting the possibilities of feeling-in-the-world from a-body. And that, in confinement, allowed people to reconnect with others, with co-living, reproducing the social bond that modifies nature to make it a body and that builds commensality as the only human way of eating.

References

Aguirre, P., Díaz Córdova, D. & y Polischer, G. (2015). *Cocinar y comer en Argentina hoy.* Buenos Aires: Fundasap y Sociedad Argentina de Pediatría. [*Cook and eat in Argentina today*. Buenos Aires: Fundasap and Argentine Society of Pediatrics]. ISBN: 978-987-1279-23-4.

Boragnio, A. (2020ª). ¿Qué comen las mujeres trabajadoras de oficina? Prácticas del comer de mujeres empleadas de la Administración Pública Nacional. *Estudios Sociales, Revista de Alimentación Contemporánea y Desarrollo Regional*, N°56 (31). [What do women office workers eat? Eating practices of women employed by the National Public Administration. *Social Studies, Journal of Contemporary Food and Regional Development*, N°56 (31)]. https://www.ciad.mx/estudiosociales/index.php/es/article/view/891.

Boragnio, A. (2020b). Producción de subjetividades en el autocuidado alimentario cotidiano. En Epele, M. y Del Mónaco (Comp.) *Tecnologías y Técnicas en Investigaciones de la Salud.* Buenos Aires: Estudios Sociológicos Editora. [Production of subjectivities in daily food self-care. In Epele, M. and Del Mónaco (Comp.) *Technologies and Techniques in Health Research.* Buenos Aires: Sociological Studies Editor].

Boragnio, A. y Sordini, V. (2019). Gustos y prácticas alimentarias de mujeres empleadas de oficinas públicas y mujeres destinatarias de programas alimentarios en Argentina. *Aposta. Revista de Ciencias Sociales*. N°81, abril, mayo y junio 2019. [Tastes and food practices of women employees of public offices and women recipients of food programs in Argentina. *Aposta. Journal of Social Sciences.* N°81, April, May and June 2019]. ISSN 1696-7348. pp. 69-86.

Contreras Hernández, J. (2005). La modernidad alimentaria. Entre la sobreabundancia y la inseguridad. *Revista Internacional de Sociología (RIS)*, Tercera Época, N°40, Enero-Abril, 2005, pp. 109-132. [Food modernity. Between overabundance and insecurity. *International Journal of Sociology (RIS)*, Tercera Época, N°40, January-April, 2005, pp. 109-132].

Fernández-Armesto, F. (2009). *Historia de la comida. Alimentos, cocina y civilización*. Barcelona: Tusquets Editores. [*History of food. Food, cuisine and civilization*. Barcelona: Tusquets Editores].

Fischler, C. (1995). *El (h)omnívoro. El gusto, la cocina y el cuerpo.* Barcelona: Anagrama. [*The (h)omnivore. The taste, the kitchen and the body.* Barcelona: Anagram].

Fischler, C. (2010). Gastro-nomía y gastro-anomía. Sabiduría del cuerpo y crisis biocultural de la alimentación moderna. *Gazeta de Antropología.* N°26. ISSN 0214-7564-222. [Gastro-nomia and gastro-anomy. Wisdom of the body and biocultural crisis of modern food. *Gazeta de Antropología*. N°26. ISSN 0214-7564-222].

García, L. J. (2013). *Una historia comestible. Homínidos, cocina, cultura y ecología.* Gijón: Ediciones TREA. [*An edible story. Hominids, cuisine, culture and ecology.* Gijón: TREA Editions].

Mintz, S. (1996). *Dulzura y poder. El lugar del azúcar en la historia moderna.* Siglo XXI Editores, México. [*Sweetness and power. The place of sugar in modern history.* Siglo XXI Editores, Mexico].

Pérez, J. A. y De Ávila, M. (2011, abril 25-29). *El anillo de cobordismo de Thom.* Escuela de Primavera de Matemáticas. Universidad Autónoma de Zacatecas, abril de 2011. *Cursos.*, Vol. *1*, (2012). Publicaciones Electrónicas Sociedad Matemática Mexicana. [*Thom's cobordism ring.* Spring School of Mathematics, Autonomous University of Zacatecas, April 2011. Courses. Vol. 1 (2012). Electronic Publications Mexican Mathematical Society.] http://www.pesmm.org.mx/ Serie%20Cursos _archivos/PCU1_1.pdf.

Poulain, J. P. (2002). *Sociologies de l 'alimentation.* París: Presses Universitaires de France. [*Sociologies of Food.* París: Presses Universitaires de France].

Scribano, A. (2007). La sociedad hecha callo: conflictividad, dolor social y regulación de las sensaciones. En Scribano, A. (comp.) *Mapeando interiores. Cuerpo, conflicto y sensaciones.* Córdoba: Jorge Sarmiento Editor. [Society shut down: conflict, social pain and regulation of sensations. In Scribano, A. (comp.) *Mapping interiors. Body, conflict and sensations.* Córdoba: Jorge Sarmiento Editor].

Scribano, A. (2012). Sociología de los cuerpos/emociones. *Revista Latinoamericana de Estudios sobre Cuerpos, Emociones y Sociedad - RELACES.* N°10. Año 4. Diciembre 2012-marzo de 2013. Córdoba. ISSN: 1852.8759. pp. 93-113. [Sociology of bodies/emotions. *Latin American Journal of Studies on Bodies, Emotions and Society - RELACES.* N°10. Year 4. December 2012-March 2013. Córdoba.

ISSN: 1852.8759. pp. 93-113.] http://www.relaces.com.ar/index.php/relaces/article/view/224.

Scribano, A. (2015). Una aproximación al estado de las sensibilidades en Argentina desde la(s) Politica(s) de la Perversión. En Sanchez Aguirre, R. (comp.) *Sentidos y sensibilidades: exploraciones sociológicas sobre cuerpos/emociones.* Buenos Aires: Estudios Sociológicos Editora. [An approach to the state of sensitivities in Argentina from the Policy(s) of Perversion. In Sanchez Aguirre, R. (comp.) *Senses and sensibilities: sociological explorations on bodies/emotions.* Buenos Aires: Sociological Studies Editora].

Scribano, A. (2018). Emotion, space, and society: a language of sensibilities (in press).

Von Scheve, C. & Jan Slaby, J. (2019). Emotion, emotion concept. Forthcoming in: Slaby, J. & von Scheve, C. (eds.) *Affective Societies: Key Concepts*. New York: Routledge.

Wiley & Sons Aubin, D. (2004). Forms of Explanations in the Catastrophe Theory of René Thom: Topology, Morphogenesis, and Structuralism. In Wise, M. N. (Ed.) *Growing Explanations: Historical Perspective on the Sciences of Complexity*. Durham: Duke University Press.

In: Emotionality of COVID-19 ISBN: 978-1-53619-534-7
Editors: M. Korstanje and S. Adrian © 2021 Nova Science Publishers, Inc.

Chapter 9

Die Alone in Argentina: A View from Sensibilities in Times of the Pandemic

Adrián Scribano[1,*] ***and Jorge Duperré***[2,†]
[1]CONICET, Argentina
[2]Universidad de Palermo, Buenos Aires, Argentina

Abstract

The objective of this work is to reflect on the sensibilities related to dying and death, in the context of the current coronavirus pandemic. The presentational strategy that we have envisaged in this regard begins by defining and establishing the theoretical perspective in which our proposal is framed: the sociology of bodies/emotions. Then we go back to another global crisis that occurred a century ago, known as the Spanish Flu. The reason for this is to recover some antecedents that allow us to enrich our approach to this phenomenon that is still ongoing; not in comparable terms (since both episodes are not), but rather illustrative.

* Corresponding Author's E-mail: adrianscribano@gmail.com. https://orcid.org/0000-0002-0523-8056.
† Corresponding Author's E-mail: jlduperre@gmail.com. https://orcid.org/0000-0003-3275-9823.

Finally, we will deal with the three traits that, in our opinion, characterize the collective bond with the dying and corpses at the present moment: mediated death, regulated death, and cherished death.

1. Introduction

The pandemic (and its management) implies a politics of sensibilities that has at least three relevant characteristics for what we want to illustrate here: a) a geometry of bodies where the proximity and distance between human beings is re-structured around the medical gaze on the healthy/sick, b) a grammar of action where the definition of who the other is operates from the denial of physical contact and c) the redefinition of the ghosts and fantasies associated with the threat of death (Scribano 2020, Scribano and De Sena 2020). Having pointed out the above, we must recognize that we are witnessing a time when all horizons of comprehensibility and expectations become strange, opaque. Policies of distancing and preventive control alter the dynamics of social interaction, public space appears alien and threatening, and public and private institutions try, in their own way, to adapt to the challenges presented by this uncertain situation[1]. Meanwhile, in the academic sphere, numerous experts are quick to characterize the current crisis as a *total social fact*, thus dusting off the analytical category that Marcel Mauss coined almost a century ago - such is the magnitude and severity of the pandemic disease, caused by the COVID-19 coronavirus. As it could not be otherwise, the catastrophe was able to acquire public notoriety as the number of deaths increased throughout the world. Just to name a few cases: on the occasion of approaching 100,000 US fatalities

[1] Even the language itself has been affected by this unique situation. And it is that, for some time now, countless neologisms related to the disease have populated everyday speech. To cite just a few cases: the "zoompleaño" is a form of celebration mediated by technological devices, which has become popular during confinement; "Infodemic" is the term with which the World Health Organization (WHO) designates the massification of false or imprecise news that circulates through the media and social networks; the verb "quarantine" has to do with the voluntary action of remaining isolated; "Coronials" refers to the generation that will be born from now on. For more information on this, visit the following *website*: https://www.clarin.com/cultura/covidiota-zoompleanos-coronials-nuevas-palabras-trae-coronavirus_0_f3apTlQiP.html

from the pandemic, the prestigious American newspaper *The New York Times* published, on its cover on Sunday, May 24, a list with the names of a thousand of them, accompanied by the following reflection: "They weren't just names on a list, they were us"[2]. Exactly two weeks earlier, the similarly prestigious Brazilian morning newspaper *O'Globo* had done something very similar, as a way of paying tribute to the 10,000 lives that COVID-19 had claimed so far in the country[3]. And the newspaper *ABC de España* denounced, on September 13, that the real death figures were double the official figures (53,000 compared to the 26,000 reported). The design chosen for this cover highlights the difference between the two figures, which are framed by drawings of hundreds of identical tombstones[4]. The funeral notices, for their part, witnessed how the death rate soared in the most affected cities. Such is the case of the newspaper *L'Eco di Bérgamo* (an Italian city in the Lombardy region), which, at the beginning of February, allocated only a page and a half to the obituaries, and a month later that section had reached 10 pages[5], or *The Boston Globe*, which went from a Sunday average of seven pages to 21 on April 26[6].

No one can foresee what political and social order will ensue. The truth is that life will not pass in the same way; neither will death and dying. Aware of how problematic it is to analyze a phenomenon still in the making –whose human and material losses are impossible to foresee in the long term– we have resorted to a precedent that, although not comparable to the present situation, gives us some keys to understand the social implications of the management of death and the dead in the context of a pandemic. We refer to that episode baptized by history as the Spanish Flu,

---

[2] To read more about this, go to: https://www.nytimes.com/es/2020/05/23/espanol/portada-NYT-coronavirus-victimas.html

[3] The title of the note is "The stories behind the Covid-19 numbers", and it is available at: https://oglobo.globo.com/sociedade/coronavirus/as-historias-por-tras-dos-numeros-da-covid-19-24419061

[4] To read more about it, go to: https://www.infobae.com/america/mundo/2020/09/13/el-diario-abc-denuncio-que-son-53000-los-muertos-por-coronavirus -en-espana-24000-mas-que-los-informados-oficial/

[5] To read more about it, go to: https://www.clarin.com/viste/coronavirus-italia-avisos-funebres-multiplican-miles_0_nNDh9hNWh. html

[6] To read more about it, go to: https://www.bostonglobe.com/2020/04/26/nation/sundays-boston-globe-runs-21-pages-death-notices-coronavirus-continues-claim-lives/

which would claim around 50 million lives across the planet in a short period of time (1918-1920).

But before entering into the problematic that summons us, we consider it necessary to make explicit the theoretical perspective from which we make our approach, namely: a sociology focused on *sensibilities*. By virtue of this, we will briefly review the theoretical-methodological and epistemological postulates on which it is based, and the centrality that the corporal/affective dimension acquires in this framework, as a fundamental indicator for the study of social structuring processes.

Once these guidelines are provided, we begin to analyze the three contingent traits that, in our opinion, make the transformations of behavior in the face of current dismissal and separation disruptive. Let us review each of them: a) a relative accentuation of that confining tendency (*ethos* of "*homo clausus* Hospitable") and desacralizing (*ethos* of the "*homo luctuosus* Secular"), noted by Norbert Elias (2009), regarding the way in which, on the one hand, the dying person is compelled to spend their last hours, and, on the other, is cremated when dead. This is a tendency that finds, in the interaction mediated by technological devices, certain mitigating factors; b) the abrupt alteration of the standardized practices of treatment and disposition of the corpse, as a result of the appearance of new mortuary dispositions, which directly affect the health system and the funeral market; and c) the debate on "bad death" and "good death", which puts the accent on the dignity of the suffering or deceased and, simultaneously, certain prevention campaigns whose "insolent" narratives update rhetoric typical of the grotesque, which come to question certain values traditionally associated with farewell rites.

We consider that these three traits - "mediated death", "regulated death" and "reverent/irreverent death" - suggest possible plots about bodily distancing (the dying person, and then his remains, as an agent of contagion) and emotional expressiveness (the socialization of pain forbidden), which are symptomatic of the present moment; these are plots that - and this is where our working hypothesis lies - would show how sensibilities around human death are reconfigured in this context of humanitarian crisis.

2. Our Theoretical Perspective

In a broad sense it is necessary here to make some clarifications aimed at explaining some starting points about a sociology of sensibilities (Scribano 2017, Scribano 2018). We consider that humans know, build and rebuild the world in and through our bodies and emotions. The most elemental form of alluded contact is the social construction of the connections between perceptions, sensations, and emotions: this builds a tripod that allows us to understand where sensibilities are founded. Thus, a set of impressions impact in the ways that subjects "exchange" with the socio-environmental context. Such impressions of objects, phenomenon, processes and other agents structure the perceptions that subjects accumulate and reproduce. Perception, from this perspective, constitutes a naturalized way of organizing the set of impressions that are given in an agent.

This weaving of impressions configures the sensations that "produce" what can be called the internal and external world: social, subjective and "natural" worlds. Such configurations are formed in a dialectic tension between impressions, perceptions and their results, that give sensations the "meaning" of a surplus or excess. Therefore, it puts them closer and beyond such dialectic. Sensations, as a result and as antecedent of perceptions, locate emotions as an effect of the processes of adjudication and correspondence between perceptions and sensations. Emotions, understood as the consequences of sensations, can be seen as a puzzle that becomes action and effect of feeling something or feeling oneself. Emotions are rooted in the "state of feeling" the world that allows the sustaining of perceptions. These are associated with socially constructed forms of sensations.

At the same time, organic and social senses also enable what seems unique and unrepeatable, as are individual sensations, and elaborate the "un-perceived work" of incorporating social elements turned into emotions. Sensations, as a result and antecedent of perceptions, give way to emotions which can be seen as the manifestation of the action and effect of feelings. They are rooted in the states of feeling the world that build perceptions associated with socially constructed forms of sensations.

Consequently, the politics of bodies (i.e., the strategies that a society accepts in order to offer a response to the social availability of individuals) is a chapter –and not the least important chapter– in the instruction manual of power. These strategies are tied and 'strengthened' by the politics of emotions that tend to regulate the construction of social sensibility.

Politics of emotions require regulating and making bearable the conditions under which social order is produced and reproduced. In this context, we understand that social bearability mechanisms are structured around a set of practices that have become embodied and that are oriented towards a systematic avoidance of social conflict.

The forms of sociability and experience are strained and twisted as if contained in a Moebius strip along with the sensibilities that arise from regulatory devices and the aforementioned mechanisms. The need to distinguish and link the possible relations between sociability, experience and social sensibilities becomes crucial at this point. Sociability is a way of expressing the means by which agents live and coexist interactively. Experience is a way of expressing the meaning gained while being in physical proximity with others, as a result of experiencing the dialogue between the individual body, the social body, and the subjective body, on the one hand; and the natural appropriation of bodily and social energies on the other. For the body to be able to reproduce experience and sociability, it is necessary that bodily energy is an object of production and consumption. Such energy can be understood as the necessary force to preserve the state of 'natural' affairs in a systemic functioning. At the same time, the social energy shown through the social body is based on bodily energy, and refers to the allocation processes of such energy as the basis of the conditions of movement and action. Thus, sensations are distributed according to the specific forms of bodily capital; and the body's impact on sociability and experience shows a distinction between the body of appearance, body of flesh, and body of movement.

Social sensibilities are continually updating the emotional schemes that arise from the accepted and acceptable norms of sensations. They are just a little long or short of the interrelationships between sociability and experience. Sensibilities are shaped and reshaped by contingent and structural overlaps of diverse forms of connection/disconnection among various ways of producing and reproducing the policies of the body and the emotions.

The politics of sensibilities are understood as the set of cognitive-affective social practices tending to the production, management and reproduction of horizons of action, disposition and cognition. These horizons refer to: 1) the organization of daily life (day-to-day, vigil/sleep, food/abstinence, etc.); 2) information to sort preferences and values (adequate/inadequate, acceptable/unacceptable, bearable/unbearable); and 3) parameters for time/space management (displacement/location, walls/bridges; enjoyment).

In this context the pandemic is itself an alteration to the policics of sensibilities and in this context of how we live death; on this we offer some considerations in the following sections.

3. The Spanish Flu as an Antecedent

All pandemics have a high social component in their genesis, reproduction and management, as Henao-Kaffur and Hernández-Álvarez (2017) say in the case of the "Spanish flu", a feature that impacts is the suddenness of deaths and the volume of them.

A feature that "death management" shares with "epidemic management" for both the Spanish Flu and COVID-19 is the isolation they produce, as summarized by Mejías Estévez, Domínguez Álvarez and Blanco Reina (2018), regarding that catastrophe at the beginning of the 20th century:

> The tragedy of this pandemic went beyond direct deaths. Fear seized the population, causing dramatic situations such as social isolation and the stigmatization of the disease. People were absent from their jobs (they did not dare to leave home), producing a direct and disastrous effect on

> the economy. In some places the authorities declared a quarantine, prohibited the right of assembly to avoid crowds, schools, theaters, centers of worship were closed ... to the point that numerous deaths of children were due to hunger (they were isolated to the point prohibiting bringing them food). (p. 665)

In this section we want to refer to how the disposition of the dead was treated in the aforementioned pandemic, as a precedent of what has happened in the case of COVID-19. It is obvious that we only undertake this in an attempt to make evident some axes of possible inquiry, but also to suggest that it is feasible to analyze similar phenomena in other times.

The British military doctor Roy Grist, who was attending Devens Camp, northwest of Boston (USA), offers the following description:

> ... we have lost many doctors and nurses ... special trains are needed to transport the dead. For several days there were not enough coffins and it was necessary to pile up the dead. A large barrack has been vacated to adapt it as a morgue ... where the corpses rest in double file ... (Roy Grist, in Murrillo Godines 2011: 463)

A central problem is the space to deposit, bury and incinerate the corpses, their transfer, and their isolation. In special areas, cities and regions in a pandemic situation must manage lifeless bodies and thereby inaugurate differential and unequal body geometries. For the same spatio-temporal context, González Bombardiere (2007) states that:

> When mortality rose to 500, 600 and 800 deaths per day, the corpses began to accumulate, there were not enough funeral homes or gravediggers, and fewer coffins. People refused to bury the dead from influenza for fear of contagion. (p. 42)

The dead and fear as a sign of the pandemic and its effects are associated with a grammar of the action of burial as a specific undertaking. All cultures have developed specific roles for those in charge of conditioning, transporting and burying their dead, practices that are modified in a pandemic: since they are not enough, given the large number of deaths. Without coffins and without sufficient gravediggers, the structure of roles and positions is modified.

Regarding the Argentine case, Adrian Carbonetti (2010) has written:

> The measures taken by the State tended to harden in November of the same year: congregations and assistance to cemeteries were suspended on the day of the dead (...) The provisions they were different in each district; thus, in the case of the province of La Rioja, these reached extremes such as the prohibition of attending wakes, except for the bereaved (p. 172)

Another modification that occurs in the Spanish Flu is that of ritual practices, which in turn, impact on the politics of the sensibilities associated with grief. The prohibition on attending cemeteries and wakes (except for the bereaved) is a clear sign of the objective difficulty of producing the practices of feeling associated with mourning and the public expression of pain. These factors end up having an impact on the social, in terms of emotional disorientation, given the key place for social affective reproduction that these practices have for society as a whole.

When Márquez Morfín and Molina del Villar (2010) analyze what happened in Mexico City, they maintain that:

> In the General Hospital, 43 had already died out of an admission of 200 patients. Due to the large number of deaths, a ditch was being opened near the Pantheon from Santa Paula, where bodies had been buried during a cholera epidemic in the mid-19th century. (p. 142)

Another basic component of burial, at least in the emotional geocultures mentioned here, is the double loss that common graves produce: the loss of a loved one and the loss of their identity among many. Again, the mechanism of grief is altered, to which is added that of memory and the personal memory of those who have been lost. In her doctoral thesis María Isabel Porras Gallo (1994) entitled "A City in Crisis: the

1918-19 flu epidemic in Madrid", makes the following components of the Spanish fever visible in the Spanish capital:

> But the difficulties for citizens did not end when they died after being struck by the flu. The problems then arose at other levels: there was a shortage of vehicles to transport the corpses to the cemeteries; coffins were sometimes missing; new cemeteries had to be set up; and it was necessary to suspend religious ceremonies and any sign proper to burials. (pp. 89-90)

And later she adds that:

> It is important to highlight that, although part of the Madrid population had health care through the medicine, burial and pharmacy societies, a very large population of Madrid had to go to the Private or public charity to receive medical assistance. (p. 164)

The situation in Madrid corroborates what has been described for Argentina and Mexico, emphatically pointing out the connection between the pandemic, the health system, the state and social position. The pandemic is a matter of state that puts the magnifying glass on the constitutive inequality of a system that denies itself as enclosed. In the same way as yesterday or today, the question arises: in what type of social structure did the pandemic appear? It is relevant for the structuring of resignation as a basic citizen emotion that will continue to this day in its "subsiadiano[7]" form (Scribano, 2019).

Finally, it is very interesting to notice the news about the flu published in the *Rif Telegram* on June 11 of 1919, that Daniel Castrillejo Pérez (2019) reproduces in his article "The 'Spanish' flu pandemic of 1918-1920. Analysis of mortality in Melilla":

> THE FLU SPREADS

[7] The expression in Spanish that refers to the union of subsidized and citizen as a new modulation of the relationship of people with the state is maintained here.

4. Healthy Measures by the Authorities

> The flu epidemic has made its appearance again in Melilla and its territory with the same intensity as last winter.
>
> Many cases are recorded daily, some with dire consequences.
>
> In hospitals, nursing has increased in a disturbing way in the last week.
>
> The Deputy Inspector of Health has brought what is happening to the knowledge of the Commander General, and in anticipation of greater evils, he has ordered the hygiene measures adopted last year to be put into effect again, relative to the permanence of the corpses in the houses, persons who must attend the funerals and careers that they must follow.
>
> Disinfection of the closed premises, of great attendance, will be carried out, and the provisions regarding the collection of garbage from homes will be taken into account.
>
> As can be seen, the authorities are not careless in the performance of their duty. Now it requires that the neighborhood not stop lending its assistance to the health work that circumstances advise.
>
> We will very much celebrate that the causes that motivate these measures disappear as soon as possible. (As cited in Castrillejo Pérez, D., 2019: 135)

The persistence of death management policies in African Spain clearly indicates that the "overflow" of societal mechanisms to administer, prepare, transport and dispose of dead bodies is a feature of the Spanish Flu that helps us to understand what happened 100 years later with COVID-19.

5. Death and Dying in Absentia

Let us now turn to the first of the traits that characterize today's dying and death: the experience experienced in a mediated way. To chart the terms in which we think about this phenomenon, we can refer to an event that took place in Milan (Italy), in mid-March. At that time, this and other cities in the country were going through one of the most pressing periods of the health emergency: massive contagion, collapsed hospitals and cemeteries. It was then that a councilor from the Democratic Party, along with other members of that group, promoted a suggestive project consisting of the donation of *tablets* to terminally ill patients, in order to alleviate the anguish caused by spending their last days in absolute solitude[8]. Under the slogan "the right to say goodbye", the group headed by Lorenzo Musotto made it possible for patients who had been admitted to an intensive care unit (IDU) to communicate for the last time with their families, through video calls. In his Facebook account, the councilor stated that: "The idea of not being able to say goodbye hurts me more than death itself [...] I know of the importance of masks, gloves and medical instruments, but the right to say goodbye, for the who leave and for those who stay, it should not be less ". It is noted here that the affective bond is of the same importance as health care. At this point, a characteristic feature of the COVID-19 pandemic can be observed: the transformations in the goodbyes, in the last goodbyes, point in the direction of an awareness of a reflective act on the meeting, on the co-presence (*sensu* Giddens). Consumer capitalism, societies normalized in acts of immediate enjoyment, the vertigo of a society thrown into the accumulation and depredation of the planet put aside, put in parentheses, did not give importance to the fact that all these activities were given by the encounter, for the accompaniment. The pandemic interrupts noise, speed and demands a new redefinition of the encounter with others, and very radically so about the last encounter; death challenges us to think of life as always. In this direction, it can be argued that, by investigating how societies deal with death, there are clues to the way in which these societies define encounters. Death in the context of COVID-19 becomes a demand due to the urgency of redefining what is everyday unthought in co-presence.

With regard strictly to mortuary rites, in our country there have been services for a few years that allow non-participation *in-praesentiain* the farewell of the deceased; an alternative that, in these circumstances, is

---

[8] To read more about it, go to: https://www.infobae.com/america/mundo/2020/03/18/el-derecho-a-decir-adios-la-donacion-que-conmueve-a-italia/

worthwhile. Among them, we highlight the one provided by two companies: a) Almavis[9] (a compound word that combines the terms "soul" and "notice") from the Province of Córdoba. According to what it announces on its website, it deals with providing "technological solutions" to the local and national funeral sector, specifically in everything that has to do with "multimedia condolences." Among the tools they sell are: the "Virtual Cemetery" (a place relatives can access to view the profile of the deceased, upload content in different formats, leave greetings, etc.), the "Smart Module" (a screen with a Wi-Fi connection that plays the messages sent by the bereaved while the wake is being held), a "mobile app" (through which funeral notices from the town specified by the user are received) and the "Plaque with code" (a device that is placed on the tombstones in order for visitors to share a message, condolences or words to relatives in the profile of the deceased; b) Grupo Pieve[10], from the Province of Salta, offers the option of "Wake online", that is: "follow the wake of your loved one if he is outside the province or the country through the cameras that are located in our Wake-Up rooms and we also have a PC so that you can communicate through a video conference with the person you want to accompany."

Similar services are provided by other companies such as the Previnca Group of the Province of Santa Fe or Previsora del Paraná, which has branches in numerous cities in Corrientes, Chaco, Misiones and Formosa. One aspect that appears frequently in all its advertisements in this regard is the importance of the human bond (although not *in absentia*), to face the anguish generated by the death of a "loved one".

Virtual obituaries (inheritors of the traditional funeral notices that even today have a specific section in the written press), are nothing new in the mortuary category, but today they acquire greater visibility with the sophistication of ICT and the expansion of social networks. In such a way, nowadays, the relatives have countless interactive tools for the commemoration of their loved one (greetings, reminders, events, etc.). To

---

[9] The mission of the firm is: "to revalue the services provided at the moment the mourning process begins". Website: http://almavis.com.ar/nosotros

[10] In the "Grief" "tab", the client finds several "useful tips" to better cope with a "loss". Website: http://www.grupopieve.com/sepelios.html

cite just one example, some firms promote candles and virtual flower arrangements, which clients can light and/or give away (symbolically), as an additional way of honoring the deceased. In the specific case of social networks, Facebook, for example, allows people close to a deceased user to manage their account to receive condolences, reminders, thanks and other communications.

Circumstantially (or not), the "Social, Preventive and Compulsory Isolation" –decreed by the Argentine government in March, and still in force in much of the national territory–, has radically changed the way we conduct ourselves before the dying and deceased. By virtue of this, legal, business and hygienic discourses –which knew how to permeate moral and affective imperatives at death and after, or preventive/palliative logics– seem more ancient than ever. In this framework, technological devices would contribute, to some extent, to suture the disunity resulting from this new "body geometry" (Scribano, 2007), and thereby attenuate the emotions generated by not being with (or feeling) who "is just gone" or will soon be.

In this context, one of the most interesting and important "concerns" of preventive isolation is generated, referring to the impossibility of witnessing death and therefore the impossibility of living it, since we live death through the death of the others. Beyond the sadness, pain or indignation that the death of a loved one can cause, not being able to live it makes it impossible to go through grief in the way that our society has long designed and designated this process. In this case, two moments of the same process converge related to not being able to be next to each other, and not being able to live death through the other. On the one hand, it appears to us as an impossibility of accompaniment and, on the other, as an impossibility of saying farewell. Accompaniment and farewell constitute the central axes of our relationship with death; a measure of health policy turned into a thanato-political strategy that involves the anguish and anxieties associated with the experience of death.

6. The Dangerousness of the Corpse: How to Proceed

In line with the previous point, we have been able to survey a set of provisions that Argentine national, provincial and municipal authorities have recently promulgated on preventive matters. Among them, we distinguish, due to the nature of their prescriptions, two regulations published on last April 23rd: a) "COVID 19. Recommendations for the Management of Corpses", of the Ministry of Health of the Nation (MSN); and b) the "Procedure for the Management of Corpses of COVID-19 Cases"[11], from the homonymous portfolio of the Government of the Autonomous City of Buenos Aires (MSGCABA). Let's review some points that are of particular importance for our analysis:

As anticipated in their titles, documents do not have the status of a mandatory compliance standard; they are, rather, recommendations or suggestions regarding how to proceed in the face of an inanimate body suspected of infection. The reason for this is the lack of information on, for example, the risk of contagion from the corpse and how long this risk may last. This is how the texts express it, in their introductory parts:

> There is currently no specific guide for the management of corpses of people who have died from COVID-19, but the provisions of the published World Health Organization Guidelines may apply. in 2014 on Prevention and control of acute respiratory infections with epidemic and pandemic tendencies during health care ... (MSN: 1)
>
> Notwithstanding that, to date, the existence of a risk of infection from corpses has not been solidly evidenced of people killed by COVID-19, in accordance with the precautionary principle and what is observed for other viruses that affect the respiratory tract, it is considered that the corpses could pose a risk of infection for people who come into direct contact with them (MSGCABA: 4)

---

[11] The Buenos Aires government clarifies that the prescriptions included in this document complement the "Protocol for the treatment of corpses, stillbirths, segments and anatomical parts in GCBA hospitals", approved in 2014, and in force to date. This material is available at: https://www.buenosaires.gob.ar/sites/gcaba/files/protocolo.pdf

As a result of these conjectures, the authorities suggest that health and funeral personnel reduce the tasks related to the treatment, transfer and disposal of the eventually infected corpse to the minimum (respecting, they add, the "human dignity" attributed to the deceased person, and the diversity of rites and creeds professed by the deceased[12]). In addition to autopsies, it is recommended to avoid "cleaning actions" and conservation (thanatopraxy) and cosmetic (thanatoesthetic) practices. Thus, a central axis of the relationship between the pandemic and death is revealed: the body as a witness to the potency of the virus, the threat of the virus, and the brand of the virus for the future. It can be clearly seen how the connection between aesthetics and politics takes a dramatic turn: presenting the body is already a risk and death is once again killed, since, if death separates the living from the dead, this is a form of death that separates the dead.

The custom of holding a wake is also discouraged, in order to prevent the crowding of people in closed spaces and the exposure of the deceased to an "open box". What is contemplated is the following:

> Prior to the transfer of the body, with a probable or confirmed cause of death by COVID.19, the personnel in charge and with medical criteria, may only authorize a direct relative and/or legal representative with authorization judicial (spouse, partner, children, parents), access to the isolation room in the hospital environment [...] All physical contact with the body and/or material surfaces that were around them is prohibited ". (MSGCABA: 6)

It is necessary to clarify that, before these recommendations were made public, most of the country's funeral companies had already implemented some prevention measures, which included precisely the limitation of the assistance offered to relatives in relation to funerals and

---

[12] In relation to the religious precepts on the fate of human remains, the controversy generated by the cremation, by prescription of the health authorities of the Province of Chaco, of a member of the Jewish community, in the framework of the pandemic of coronavirus disease. For more details, consult the article "Creation controversy unleashes the first Jewish deceased by COVID-19 in Argentina" (Jewish Link, 03/29/20). Available at: https://www.enlacejudio.com/2020/03/29/desata-controversia-cremacion-del-primer-judio-fallecido-por-covid-19-en-argentina/.

other honors.[13] We were able to verify this from a partial survey of the institutional portals that these companies have on the Internet. In order to conduct the search and make the systematization of the information more operational, we decided to limit the survey to those firms that are part of the "Argentine Federation of Funeral and Related Services Entities" (Fadedsfya)[14]. Of the total number of web pages (56), we found a dozen burial houses that inform the public about the preventive measures they have taken as a result of the pandemic. Let's look at some examples:

The Parque San Agustín company, which has branches in various towns in Tucumán, accompanies the notice of closure of its offices with the slogan "In the distance closer than ever"[15]. For its part, the San Bernardo Sepelios company[16], located in the same province, shares a series of recommendations on how to deal with grief in isolation. To mention only one of them:

> Recommendations for the care of the bereavement of the quarantined child [...] since in that case the children will not have the opportunity to visit [their grandfather or grandmother], or to show them affection such as kisses or hugs [...] it is recommended that parents suggest that their children write a letter, send a message or make video calls by phone to a loved one who is ill, to alleviate to a certain extent the impossibility of offering them signs of affection in person [...] given the impossibility of celebrating funeral rites due to confinement measures [parents are recommended] to propose to the child to carry out some symbolic activity [...] such as drawing a picture, writing a letter or choosing a photograph of themselves ...

---

[13] The reason for the early adoption of these internal provisions had to do, among other things, with the contagion registered in a burial house in the San Martín district (Greater Buenos Aires). The incident occurred at the beginning of April, when the funeral home received the body of a woman from a health center. Those responsible for it allegedly omitted the true causes of death (which led to a criminal case for negligence). As a result, two funeral agents were infected, as well as relatives of the deceased and clinic staff. For more information, visit the following portal *web*: www.filo.news/actualidad/Duenos-de-una-cocheria-se-contagiaron-de-coronavirus-de-un-cuerpo-infectado-20200417-0003.html

[14] The other organization that completes the national picture is the "Argentine Federation of Funeral Associations" (Fadaf). Website: www.fadaf.org.ar

[15] Website: https://www.parquesanagustin.com.ar/noticia/66/informacion-importante-oficina

[16] Website: http://www.sanbernardosepelios.com.ar/

At the regional level, the impact of the health crisis has intensified. The scenes of bodies scattered through the streets of Guayaquil, of mass burials in the Vila Formosa de San Pablo cemetery (the largest in Latin America), or of the "humanitarian command for the removal of corpses" that daily travel the streets of Lima, corroborate the diagnosis made by the World Health Organization in May, regarding that "South America has become a new epicenter of the coronavirus"[17]. Therefore, it is not surprising that most countries are limiting all types of public acts, and funerals are no exception. The measures have been so rigorous - and their emotional consequences so damaging - that the Inter-American Commission on Human Rights (IACHR) released a statement the same month urging OAS member states to "respect and guarantee the rights of relatives of those who died in the framework of the COVID-19 pandemic, allow mortuary rites in a manner appropriate to the circumstances and, with this, contribute to the preservation of their memory and tribute."[18]

7. A Dignified and Irreverent Death

In Argentina, the norms of hospital confinement and the restriction of funerals soon caused discomfort among the families of the infected, health and funeral agents and other actors involved. Consequently, a series of protocols began to be implemented to guarantee the final accompaniment and farewell. For example, we can cite the initiative that the Rodolfo Rossi Hospital of the City of La Plata (Buenos Aires) carried out in June, called "Die accompanied"[19]. It guarantees that a family member accompanies a terminal patient with coronavirus. The interesting thing is that, in its

---

[17] To read more about this, go to: https://www.bbc.com/mundo/noticias-america-latina-52776325

[18] Press Release 097/20 of the Inter-American Commission on Human Rights (IACHR) "Respect for the mourning of the families of the people who died in the COVID-19 Pandemic." Available at: http://www.oas.org/es/cidh/prensa/comunicados/2020/097.asp

[19] To read more about this, go to: https://www.infobae.com/sociedad/2020/07/23/morir-acompanado-el-protocolo-que-implemento-un-hospital-para-que-las-muertes-By-coronavirus-don't-be-lonely/

foundations, this program affirms that "dying in company can be in itself a palliative act".

In a similar direction, at the end of August the Legislature of the City of Buenos Aires approved a law that contemplates "the right to the last goodbye", being the first jurisdiction in the country to sanction a measure with these characteristics. Among other concessions, it enables a person "from the affective environment of the patient to go to the hospital and facilitate, with a mobile device, communication with the rest of the family or relatives of the patient." Days later, the Ministry of Health published the corresponding protocol for the implementation of the law. Among its provisions, it specifies that "the companion may carry objects" of emotional value to the patient, such as photos or letters.

At the national level, the health authorities released, also in August, a set of "recommendations" not only to allow the affective bond in these critical circumstances, but also the "interdisciplinary" containment of the patient's family[20]. And they are recommendations because they address the particularities that a dismissal situation entails, in accordance with the availability of medical and psychological staff, beds, supplies, etc., but also deal with the specific emotional needs of each family; these are aspects that protocols tend to omit, argue the authors of the regulation.

In these examples becomes evident, once again, the centrality that the problem of what we call death acquires *in absentia* and how technological devices are considered as a valid alternative to manage the affective damages of separation. Even so, co-presence is an essential requirement to go through these final instances in the least traumatic way possible, as suggested by the aforementioned regulations, regarding containment between the bereaved, relatives and palliativists. Now, what has come to update the confinement of the dying and the estrangement from the deceased - whose bodies have now become vectors of contagion - is the discussion about the "good death" and the "bad death". In line with what

[20] More about these regulations at: https://www.lanacion.com.ar/sociedad/coronavirus-argentina-buscan-habilitar-ley-ciudad-acompanamiento-nid2429492 - https://www.baenegocios.com/sociedad/Como-is-the-CABA-protocol-to-visit-relatives-in-critical-state-20200826-0035.html - https://www.pagina12.com.ar/288018-coronavirus-las-recomendaciones- of-the-ministry-of-health-for

was stated by Laura Marina Panizo and Valérie Robin Azevedo (2020), we consider that the difference between both dimensions is determined not only by the causes of death, but also by the treatment given to those bodies. And the decisions made in this regard will result in a lesser or greater "pathologization" of the grief, depending on the case. Hence, those who call for the relaxation of sanitary restrictions, appeal with recurrence to the dignity of the victims of contagion and their right to be cremated in the most "humane" way possible. In this context, dignified death appears to be associated less with the claim of orthothanasia, than with the recognition of the right to jointly experience such a disturbing outcome.

At the same time that these demands acquired public status, social networks continued to be populated with countless content referring to the social emergency and its multiple effects. From testimonies of those who were directly or indirectly affected by the disease and the consequent preventive measures, to events of global impact from the four cardinal points, passing through the increasingly sophisticated *fake news*; all this production and circulation of information has also caused the sensations, perceptions and emotions related to dying and death to be challenged with unusual assiduity.

If we conceive, as Scribano and Lisdero (2018) do, that looking/showing/feeling and receiving/sharing in and through networks suppose specific ways of elaborating perceptions - and that the latter are related to affective regimes and management of sensations mediated by ICTs–, then we can recognize the importance of the question of the way in which sensibilities are structured in virtual environments. And exchanges on fatality in times of pandemic are a good starting point.

Among the profuse material in this regard, perhaps the most viralized content (worth the term) so far is the one that has as its central theme the ballad of the Ghanaian *pallbearers*: a charismatic group of funeral directors, whose jovial choreography (edited together with a catchy identifying melody) would have sufficient ductility to adapt to any risky situation –real or apparent– that arose; including, of course, the contagion of viral disease. Such has been the popularity of this meme, that it was even used for different prevention campaigns in various countries. To mention a few cases: the Republican National Guard of Portugal shared on its official account *Facebook* a photomontage in which a poster with the African protagonists appears, accompanied by the following warning: "Stay home or dance with them! What do you prefer?"[21]. Just published, the post was shared more than 2,000 times and received hundreds of comments.

The Colombian National Police, for its part, recorded a video in which they emulate that choreography, to raise awareness of the importance of confinement to the inhabitants of Quibdó (Department of Chocó)[22].

The curious thing about this phenomenon is the carefree and cheerful character with which the current crisis is approached, perhaps as a way of warding off the misery, fear and anguish caused by the daily verification of the mortality and lethality rates of COVID- 19. From our perspective, this palliative vocation would correspond to a type of affective regime with a certain preponderance in the present mediated interactions. Likewise, we suppose that the "irreverent" way of behaving in the face of dying and death in the context of a pandemic is stressed by other logics of feeling/wanting: those associated with the claim for the right to dignified treatment, dismissal and separation, which develop above.

CONCLUSION

Throughout these pages we try to reflect on the specificities, in our opinion the most relevant, that suffering/perishing acquires in the context of the current health crisis. In this sense, we base our approach on the perspective of a sociology of bodies/emotions, with the emphasis placed on the structuring of present sensibilities. The impossibility of referring to conclusive information on a phenomenon still in progress - and which, due to its magnitude and nature, does not have any contemporary referentiality

---

[21] To read more about it, go to: https://www.farodevigo.es/mundo/2020/04/17/africanos-ataud-secreto-mejor-guardado/2277242.html

[22] To read more about this, go to: https://actualidad.rt.com/actualidad/350268-policia-colombia-baila-ataud-calle-meme-africano-coronavirus

either - made us go back to the Spanish Flu (1918-1920) and the corresponding hygienic measures adopted. Specifically, we considered how the management of corpses at that time configured an unprecedented "body geometry", heralding a practice of distancing that today acquires the status of what we have called "death *in absentia*".

And it is precisely this reconfiguration of the links between the bereaved/deceased and the social environment that has influenced the tensions between different "affective regimes", which gain visibility on at least two levels: a) the regulations relating to hospital and funeral procedures, and b) the "management of sensations" in and through the networks, around the treatment of death in the times of coronavirus.

Ultimately, what it is about is a tragic event that has come to question, perhaps as never before, that politics of bodies and emotions that made the disturbing "tangibility" of the perishable more bearable.

The pandemic causes human beings to die alone; poor, rich, of all and various genders, of all ethnic groups, as in all dimensions of social structuring, the pandemic operates as a magnifying glass on the contemporary global structure: it isolates. It is precisely in the gale of volatility that death installs where the world has had to cling to love beyond all the discredit that colonial/patriarchal reason throws on that energy that breaks isolation and is therefore dangerous.

REFERENCES

Carbonetti, A. (2010) "History of a forgotten epidemic. The Spanish flu pandemic in Argentina, 1918-1919", in *Desacatos*, núm. 32, enero-abril 2010. pp. 159-174.

Castrillejo Pérez, D. (2019) "The 'Spanish' flu pandemic of 1918-1920. Melilla´s mortality analysis", in *Revista Trápana*, núm. 12, diciembre 2019. pp. 123-138.

Elias, N. (2009) *The loneliness of the dying*. México: Fondo de Cultura Económica.

González Bombardiere, S. (2007) "The forgotten pandemic of 1918", in *Ars médica, revista de estudios médicos humanísticos*, núm. 14, vol. 14 2007. pp. 39-48.

Henao-Kaffur, L. y Hernández-Álvarez, M. (2017) "The flu pandemic in 1918: A case of social subsumption of the biological in the social", in *Americanía, Revista de Estudios Latinoamericanos*. Nueva Época (Sevilla), núm. 6, julio-diciembre, 2017. pp. 8-52.

Márquez Morfín, L. y Molina Del Villar, A. (2010) "1918 autumn: the impact of the influenza pandemic in Mexico City", in *Desacatos*, núm. 32, enero-abril 2010. pp. 121-144.

Mejías Estévez, M. J., Domínguez Álvarez, R. y Blanco Reina, E. (2018) "The Influenza Pandemic in 1918: Myths and Realities from the Scientific Literature", in *Journal of Negative and No Positive Results, JONNPR*. 2018, núm. 8, vol. 3, 2018. pp. 655-673.

Ministerio de Salud del Gobierno de la Ciudad Autónoma De Buenos Aires (2020) *Procedure for Handling of Dead Bodies in COVID-19 Cases*. Buenos Aires, Argentina.

Ministerio de Salud de la Nación (2020) *COVID 19. Recommendations for Handling of Dead Bodies*. Buenos Aires, Argentina.

Murillo Godínez, G. (2011) "Remembering the Spanish flu", in *Med Int Mex*. núm. 5, vol. 27, septiembre-octubre 2011. pp. 463-466.

Panizo, L. M. y Azevedo, V. R. (2020) *Turning the "bad death" in the Covid-19 era*. Instituto Francés de Estudios Andinos. Ministre de l'Europe et des Affaires étrangères. París. https://ifea.hypotheses.org/4119

Porras Gallo, M. I. (1994) *A City in Crisis: the 1918-19 flu epidemic in Madrid*. Departamento de Salud Pública e Historia de la Ciencia. Facultad de Medicina Universidad Complutense de Madrid. https://eprints.ucm.es/2765/

Scribano, A. (2020) "The war of the curves: pandemic, sensibilities and social structuring", in *Simbiótica. Revista Eletrônica*, 7(1), 53-68. Retrieved from: http://periodicos.ufes.br/simbiotica/article/view/30982

Scribano, A. (2018) *Politics and Emotions*. Houston USA: Studium Press llc. p.240.

Scribano, A. (2017) *Normalization, enjoyment and bodies/emotions: Argentine sensibilities*. New York: Nova Science Publishers. p.236.

Scribano, A. (2007) "Health, money and love...! Stories from university students about the body and health", in *Policromía Corporal. Cuerpos, Grafías y Sociedad*, Scribano, A. (comp.), Jorge Sarmiento Editor-Universitas Libro. pp. 97-123.

Scribano, A. and de Sena, A. (2020) "The New Heroes: Applause and Sensibilities in the Era of the COVID-19", in *Culture e Studi del Sociale*, 5(1), Special issue, 273-285. http://www.cussoc.it/index.php/journal/issue/archive1.

Scribano, A. y Lisdero, P. (2018) "Visual Experience and Social Research: towards a critique of the political economy of the digital gaze", in *Religación, Revista de ciencias sociales y humanidades*, vol. 3, núm. 9, marzo 2018. Quito, Ecuador. pp. 165-181. [*Religation, Journal of Social Sciences and Humanities*]

About the Authors

Freddy Timmermann is professor at O'Higgins University, Chile. He is PhD in history and has published extensively in the fields of terrorism research. Dr. Timmermann has served as key note speakers in countless academic events and courses. His field of expertise falls in the study of fear in the 70s decade as well as the human right violation during Pinochet´s regime.

Aldana Boragnio, is Doctor in Sociology from the University of Alicante, Spain (UA). Master in Research in Social Sciences, Graduate in Sociology and Professor of Secondary, Normal and Special Education in Sociology from the University of Buenos Aires, Argentina (UBA). She is a member of the Study Group on the Sociology of Emotions and Bodies (GESEC) of the Gino Germani Research Institute (UBA) and the Center for Sociological Research and Studies (CIES). She is a researcher in the Working Group "Sensibilities, Subjectivities and Poverty" of the Latin American Council of Social Sciences (CLACSO) and co-director of the Recognition Project "Social Policies and Food Practices" of the University of Buenos Aires. She takes part of Academic Secretary of the Research Center on Consumption, Sensitivities and Creativity (CICSEC) of the

University of Palermo (UP) as well as Professor in the Social Psychology subject of the Sociology career at the University of Buenos Aires. Collaborating editor in the Latin American Journal of Studies on Bodies, Emotions and Society (RELACES). She currently holds a postdoctoral fellowship from the National Council for Scientific and Technical Research (CONICET), Argentina. Her research work focuses on emotions, eating and commensalities from the perspective of Bodies/Emotions.

Primavera Fisogni (1963), Italian philosopher and journalist, is currently editor at La Provincia daily newspaper in Como (Italy). She was educated at the Catholic University of Milan, where she graduated in classics and in theoretical philosophy. She took the PhD in metaphysics at the Pontifical University of the Holy Cross in Rome, directed by Spanish scholar Lluìs Clavell. Her essays are mainly aimed at exploring the premoral origins of evildoing (Terroristi. La persona nell'agire eversivo, 2004; L'inaridimento dei terroristi, 2009; Dehumanization and Human Fragility, 2013) and are focused on the phenomenology of dialogue (Incontro al dialogo, 2006). As a feminist thinker, she explores theoretical arguments for the female priesthood in the Catholic Church (A Love Life in a Sexless Condition, 2011). She was awarded as a reporter in 2002 and 2009. As a philosopher, she won the Prize Leggere Donna for her investigation about terrorism. She is author of DEhumanization and human fragility: a philosophical investigation, 2013 & The Good of Life 2015 (authorHouse).

Pedro Lisdero holds a bachelor's degree in Sociology (U. Siglo XXI, Córdoba, Argentina) and PhD in Social Studies of Latin America (Center for Advanced Studies—National University of Córdoba). Lisdero is a researcher at the National Scientific and Technological Research Council (CONICET, Argentina), Co-director of the Program of Studies on Collective Action and Social Conflict of the Center for Research and Studies on Cultures and Societies (CONICET and National University of

Córdoba—UNC), and a researcher at the Centre for Sociological Research and Studies (CIES, Argentina). In addition, he is an Assistant Professor and Chair of "General Sociology" at the National University of Villa Maria (UNVM), Director of Sociological Studies Editora (ESEditora—CIES), and a member of the editorial team of RELACES, RELMIS, and Onteaiken. He is also a member of the Research Centre on Consumption, Sensibilities and Creativity (CICSEC) - University of Palermo.

Marion Fonrouge, is a Psychoanalyst and Psychologist, Professor at the National University of La Plata. International Degree in Social Studies on Bodies and Emotions (CIES, Research and Sociological Studies Center). Fonrouge is a member of the Social Studies Group on Sociology of Bodies and Emotions, School of Social Sciences, Gino Germani Research Institute University of Buenos Aires, Director PhD Adrián Scribano. Member of the Research Centre on Consumption, Sensibilities and Creativity (CICSEC) - University of Palermo. Research line: Sensibilities, Consumption and Enjoyment in Freud, S. Marx, K. Lacan, and Scribano, A. perspectives, The Happiness Imperative and Enjoyment as mandatory for Capitalistic Society. Subjectivity Production: ¿Unconscious Capitalism or Capitalism Unconscious?

Irina Burak is a PhD in Economics and professor at Lomonosov Moscow State University, Russia. She was born in Moscow region on the 28th of February 1989. In 2006, Dr Burak finished school with honors and entered Lomonosov Moscow State University, Faculty of Economics. In 2012 she received a bachelor diploma with honors and a medal for excellent academic achievements while earning a diploma with the degree of "Master of Economics" in 2014. In 2018 she was awarded PhD degree in Economics. She serves as an Associate professor at Lomonosov Moscow State University, Department of Labor economics and personnel, and as a Head of Further Professional Education Department with 14+ years of experience. As author Dr Burak wrote 25 academic papers related to labor market and further professional education including publications in Web of Science journals and proceedings while taking part in scientific research, conferences and round tables on the subject of labor economics and further professional education and also give seminars on the subjects of «Labor economics» and «Personnel economics» for bachelors and «Human Resource Management» and «Organizational Behavior» for masters. Dr Burak completed 11 professional development programs including international. She has advanced level in English (London House School of English, England) and B2-level in Italian (University of Bologna, Italy). She is married and has a 3-years old daughter.

Tatiana Razumova is Doctor of Economics, professor at Lomonosov Moscow State University. She was born in Moscow on the 15th of July 1958. Dr. Razumova is graduated with honors from the Faculty of Economics of Lomonosov Moscow State University in 1980. In 2008 she was awarded the honorary title "Honorary Lecturer of the Moscow University". Now she works as a Head of Labor Economics and Personnel Chair at the Faculty of Economics (MSU) and has 36 years of scientific and pedagogical experience. Tatiana has published 125 works, including 91 scientific and 34 educational works, including publications in Web of Science journals and proceedings. Dr. Razumova conducts scientific and analytical, research and expert work. Prelects both in Russian and in English on the subjects: "Labor Economics", "Personnel Economics", "Introduction to Project Analysis", "New Forms of Employment", "Personnel Management", "Human Resources Management in International Companies", "Organizational Behavior" at different educational levels (bachelors, masters, postgraduate training programs, MBA) at the Faculty of Economics. She has extensively participated in several international, all-Russian and departmental conferences, round tables related to labor market and further professional education. Regularly takes part in professional development programs including international. Member of Dissertation Council at Lomonosov Moscow State University. Has advanced level in English. She is married and has two daughters.

Fabio La Rocca, is a sociologist, PhD of Sorbonne University of Paris and Maître de conférences at Université Paul Valéry Montpellier 3 (France) where he is a researcher at LERSEM-IRSA (Centre of research in sociology and imaginary). He teaches visual sociology, urban imaginary and ambiance, communication and pop culture. He is a member of the researcher group Kinepoliticom of the PUC-RS University of Porto Alegre (Brazil) and of the Grupo de Pesquisa CAC (Comunicação, Arte e Cidade) of the Universidade do Estado do Rio de Janeiro (FCS/UERJ). He collaborates with ATOPOS the Center Study on Digital Communication of the University of São Paulo and some university in Seoul and Pusan (Korea). He is editorial coordinator of the journal on social science *Sociétés* (Deboeck Edition). He is the author of the book *La ville dans tous ses états* (CNRS Éditions, Paris 2013, Sulina, Porto Alegre 2018) and of several articles and chapters on books with the focus on visual sociology, technologies, metropolis and images.

Angelica De Sena is a Doctor in Social Sciences from the University of Buenos Aires, she specialized in the study of Social Policies and Emotions and Methodology of Social Research. She is Independent Researcher by CONICET-UNLaM and the Gino Germani Research Institute (FCS-UBA). She coordinates the Study Group on Social Policies and Emotions at CIES (GEPSE). She is a professor in the Sociology Career, Faculty of Social Sciences, UBA. She teaches postgraduate courses at different universities in Argentina and abroad. She was visiting professor at University Cambridge, Universitá di Milano-Bicocca, Shanghai International Studies University. She is the director of the Latin American Journal of Social Research Methodology (ReLMIS). She directs research projects at UBA and UNLaM. She is the Coordinator of the UNLaM Regional Node in the Latin American Network of Social Sciences Methodology (RedMet). She is the Coordinator of the CLACSO Working Group: "Sensitivities, subjectivities and poverty". She is co-coordinator of the ISA Working Group "Society and Emotions". She participated in various scientific meetings and has published in scientific journals, book chapters and books in relation to social policies and social research methodology.

Jorge Luis Duperré earned a degree in Social Communication and is a university professor (National University of San Luis, Argentina). He is actually studying a Doctorate in Social Studies of Latin America in the National University of Córdoba, Argentina. He has published numerous works on the current problems of the *sensibilities* related to *death* and the *handling of the corpses*. His most recent titles are the remain of the death in pandemic; An Analysis of the Politics of Bodies and Contemporary Sensibilities" (2020), "Disquisitions on Death 2.0, A Study of Human Finitude in the Age of Hypermediation" (2020) and "Contemporary Ways of Signifying Human Death. From 'abject art' to Thanatosthesia" (2019)

About the Editors

Maximiliano Korstanje serves as Senior Researcher at the University of Palermo, Buenos Aires. He is Book Series Editor of *Advances in Hospitality, Tourism and Service Industries* (IGI Global, US), and *Tourism Security-Safety and Post Conflict Destinations* (Emerald Publishing, UK). In 2018, his biography was selected to be part of the roster of Alfred Nelson Marquis Lifetime Achievement Award (Marquis Who`s Who). Korstanje has also been named as Editor in Chief Emeritus for the *International Journal of Cyber-warfare and Terrorism*. Korstanje worked as Guest Professor at CERS, University of Leeds, UK, University of La Habana, Cuba & University of Las Palmas de Gran Canaria, Spain. His latest books are *Terrorism, Technology and Apocalyptic Future* (Palgrave Macmillan), *The Challenges of Democracy in the War on Terror* (Routledge) & *Tourism, Terrorism and Security* (Emerald Group Publishing).

Adrian Scribano is Senior Researcher of CONICET IIGG-FCS-UBA. Doctor of Philosophy (UBA). Degree in Development Sciences. Specialization in Political Sociology. ILADES. Santiago de Chile. Graduate in Political Science. Faculty of Political Science and International Relations. Catholic University of Córdoba. Diploma of Human Rights. Institute of Human Rights. Law School. Complutense University. Madrid. Spain. Director of the Center for Sociological Research and Studies CIES (www.estudiosociologicos.com.ar). Director of the "Latin American Journal of Studies on Bodies, Emotions and Society" (www.relaces.com.ar) Director of the "Group of Studies on Sociology of Emotions and Bodies" of the IIGG-UBA. Director of the "Study Program on Collective Action and Social Conflict (www.accioncolectiva.com.ar) registered in CEA UE CONICET (UNC) and Coordinator of "Researching Body and Emotions" (www.methodspace.com/group/researching- body-and-emotions).

INDEX

#

20th century, 16, 179
21st century, 16, 30, 143, 144, 145, 146, 149, 169

A

administrative support, 88
advertisements, 28, 66, 185
affective dimension, 74, 76, 78, 176
age, 19, 62, 86, 96, 134, 137, 153, 157, 162
ambiance, xvii, 108, 109, 201
anger, viii, 5, 133, 137
anxiety, ix, 7, 42, 69, 71, 73, 75, 91, 92, 112, 139, 140, 141, 142, 143, 144, 149, 160, 162, 167
Argentina, vi, xiv, xvii, xviii, 1, 6, 11, 12, 16, 17, 18, 19, 20, 21, 22, 23, 24, 26, 27, 29, 30, 31, 32, 33, 34, 36, 37, 59, 95, 125, 134, 136, 138, 145, 149, 151, 152, 153, 160, 161, 162, 164, 165, 166, 169, 170, 172, 173, 182, 188, 190, 194, 195, 197, 198, 201,202
armed forces, 30
Armenia, 92, 104
army, 6, 20, 21, 23, 25, 29, 32, 35
articulation, xix, 15, 30, 115, 152
artificial intelligence, 88
atmosphere, 109, 113, 115, 117
Austria, 62
authorities, 97, 99, 134, 180, 183, 187, 188, 191
awareness, 27, 28, 69, 71, 73, 74, 184, 193

B

bankruptcy, 86, 98
basic services, viii
behaviors, 42, 47, 68, 134, 142, 144, 158
Belarus, 92, 104
Belgium, 62
beneficiaries, 101, 141
benefits, 96, 104
beverages, 19
biodiversity, 118
biological processes, 15, 64
biosphere, 117
blood, 41

blood circulation, 41
bodies, xiv, 6, 11, 14, 15, 36, 37, 65, 67, 69, 79, 81, 132, 145, 146, 148, 149, 154, 155, 156, 168, 171, 172, 173, 174, 177, 180, 181, 183, 190, 191, 195, 196, 197, 199, 202, 204
bodies/emotions, 36, 81, 154, 198
body energy, 15
boredom, 7, 91, 140, 141, 144
brain, 15, 48, 79, 154
Brazil, 201
bubonic plague, 43, 44
business education, 89
business strategy, 89
businesses, 85, 98

C

call centers, 101
campaigns, 38, 176, 192
capitalism, 2, 4, 5, 8, 9, 12, 27, 65, 80, 81, 82, 119, 131, 132, 147, 184, 199
Caribbean, 16, 37
catastrophes, 12
catering, 98
central nervous system, 15, 154
children, viii, 26, 37, 85, 90, 93, 95, 96, 110, 180, 188, 189
Chile, vii, viii, ix, xi, 5, 95, 204
China, vii, xiii, 2, 9, 34, 40, 94, 95, 118
churches, ix, 20, 24, 25, 30
circulation, xv, 60, 61, 77, 192
cities, x, 2, 28, 84, 86, 108, 114, 118, 119, 135, 175, 180, 184, 185
citizens, vii, ix, 3, 6, 7, 22, 84, 96, 97, 98, 101, 103, 111, 122, 147, 182
citizenship, ix
city, xvii, 2, 7, 102, 104, 108, 109, 111, 112, 113, 114, 116, 117, 118, 119, 120, 121, 123, 126, 135, 142, 147, 175, 181, 187, 190, 191, 195
civil law, 44
civil service, 85
civilization, xi, xiii, 4, 142, 144, 147, 170
cleaning, 24, 40, 129, 188
climatic change, 119
closure, 2, 135, 189
cognition, 64, 156, 168, 169, 179
cognitive capacities, 155
cognitive dimension, 71, 78
coherence, ix, 47, 48, 50, 51
collaboration, 9, 90, 103
commensality, xviii, 8, 33, 152, 153, 154, 157, 158, 159, 164, 167, 168, 169
commodification, v, 18, 19, 59, 62, 63, 64, 66, 67, 77, 78, 79, 147
commodification of audiences, 65, 67, 78
commodity, 61, 63, 64, 66, 68, 75, 77, 80
communication, 54, 66, 80, 87, 90, 191, 201
community, x, xv, 10, 21, 26, 40, 42, 43, 45, 46, 47, 48, 49, 50, 51, 53, 64, 77, 111, 120, 123, 132, 157, 188
complement, 26, 119, 187
complexity, 53, 69, 79, 155
compliance, 21, 22, 140, 187
conception, 118, 119
conceptualization, 14, 18, 155
concern, 19, 91, 93, 139, 140, 141
conditional cash transfer programs, 18
configuration, xviii, 75, 113, 136, 142, 144, 151
confinement, xviii, 115, 151, 152, 153, 154, 164, 167, 168, 169, 174, 189, 190, 191, 193
conflict, 5, 16, 17, 22, 25, 29, 36, 40, 43, 47, 49, 50, 52, 53, 54, 142, 143, 171, 178
consciousness, 66, 67, 79
construction, 31, 62, 69, 75, 77, 89, 112, 121, 132, 144, 178
consumption, viii, x, xviii, 12, 14, 77, 81, 145, 152, 153, 158, 165, 178
contamination, xvi, 84, 115, 128
contradiction, x, 47, 53

controversial, 8, 103
cooking, xviii, 128, 152, 153, 164, 165, 167, 168
cooperation, ix, 28, 31, 99
coronavirus, xiv, xix, 10, 22, 23, 27, 33, 34, 35, 36, 38, 39, 40, 41, 44, 53, 55, 56, 69, 87, 92, 96, 97, 100, 101, 103, 104, 105, 134, 173, 174, 175, 188, 189, 190, 191, 193, 194
corpses, xix, 174, 180, 182, 183, 187, 190, 194, 202
COVID-19, v, vii, ix, x, xi, xiii, xiv, xv, xvi, xvii, 1, 2, 3, 5, 6, 7, 8, 9, 10, 11, 12, 19, 24, 26, 28, 32, 38, 39, 40, 41, 42, 43, 44, 45, 53, 56, 59, 60, 61, 62, 63, 67, 71, 72, 83, 91, 92, 94, 103, 104, 105, 108, 111, 126, 127, 130, 134, 137, 139, 140, 141, 143, 144, 152, 153, 167, 174, 175, 179, 180, 183, 184, 187, 188, 190, 195, 196
COVID-19 pandemic, x, xiv, 10, 11, 12, 19, 26, 43, 45, 53, 127, 152, 153, 184, 190
crises, 2, 16, 22
crisis management, 10
Cuba, 203
culture, 4, 8, 98, 116, 147, 157, 171, 201
Czech Republic, 62

D

danger, 3, 49, 118, 136
data analysis, 153
data center, 87
death, xiii, xiv, xix, 1, 2, 5, 8, 29, 55, 66, 121, 149, 173, 174, 175, 176, 179, 183, 185, 186, 188, 189, 190, 191, 192, 193, 194, 195, 202
death of hospitality, xiv, 1
death rate, 175
deaths, 2, 174, 179, 180, 181
decomposition, viii, ix
deficiencies, 3, 31, 133
dental practice, 98
Department of Labor, 199
depredation, 184
depth, xviii, 30, 152, 153
destruction, ix, 54, 112, 118
diet, xviii, 13, 152, 158, 165, 166, 167, 168, 169
digital affective communities, 78
digital experience, 109
digital technologies, 80
digital world, 74, 76, 80
dignity, 176, 192
diminished humanism, 30, 31
displacement, 116, 156, 179
disposition, 8, 64, 76, 114, 120, 156, 168, 169, 176, 179, 180
dissipative structure, 47
distance learning, 89, 102
distribution, 15, 19, 21, 25, 28, 94, 134, 154, 156, 169
diversification, xviii, 152
diversity, 21, 188
doctors, 27, 102, 180
dying, xix, 4, 8, 173, 175, 176, 183, 186, 191, 192, 193, 194

E

eating at home, 168
eating practices, xix, 152, 153, 157, 159, 164, 166, 167, 168, 169, 170
ecology, 115, 116, 117, 123, 171
e-commerce, 87
economic activity, 10
economic consequences, xiv, 1
economic crisis, xiii, 2, 3, 6, 16, 91, 93
economic downturn, ix
economic instability, 89
economics, x, 89, 199, 200
ecosophy, xvii, 108, 109, 115, 117, 119, 122, 123

education, ix, 9, 87, 88, 89, 98, 100, 101, 104, 105, 130, 136, 139, 141, 144, 152, 197, 200
educational attainment, 139, 141
elaboration, 25, 72, 73, 74, 76, 127, 131, 133
elderly people, xvi, 83, 100, 102
emergency, 12, 13, 17, 21, 22, 26, 33, 40, 102, 103, 120, 184, 192
emotion, 77, 136, 138, 139, 140, 141, 142, 144, 155, 165, 167, 172, 182
emotional experience, 142, 169
emotional platform, 77
emotional prosumer, 77
emotional state, 75
emotionality, 75, 118
emotions, v, vi, xiv, xv, xvii, xviii, xix, 4, 6, 7, 11, 12, 13, 14, 16, 30, 36, 59, 60, 61, 62, 64, 65, 67, 71, 72, 73, 74, 76, 77, 79, 81, 108, 110, 112, 113, 125, 126, 131, 132, 133, 134, 135, 136, 137, 138, 139, 140, 144, 145, 146, 147, 148, 149, 151, 153, 154, 155, 156, 159, 160, 162, 163, 167, 168, 169, 171, 172, 173, 177, 178, 179, 186, 192, 193, 194, 195, 196, 197, 199, 201, 204
empathy, 118
employees, 84, 85, 86, 89, 91, 96, 98, 100, 170
employment, 86, 99, 127, 129, 130
encounter, 184
energy, 13, 15, 47, 64, 77, 112, 178, 194
entertainment, 5, 8, 69, 71, 73, 74, 98, 152
entrepreneurs, 85, 98, 99, 102
environment, 14, 15, 46, 47, 48, 50, 51, 68, 113, 115, 117, 120, 121, 130, 154, 155, 156, 158, 188, 191
epidemic, xvi, 40, 44, 83, 85, 87, 99, 102, 108, 179, 181, 182, 183, 187, 194, 195
equipment, xvii, 21, 84, 88, 97, 102
exploitation, 6, 8, 65, 66, 79
expressiveness, 176
extreme poverty, 16

F

families, 17, 20, 85, 96, 184, 190
family environment, 94
family life, 158
fear, vii, ix, xi, xiv, 1, 4, 6, 7, 8, 42, 68, 69, 71, 73, 75, 87, 91, 133, 136, 138, 139, 140, 141, 142, 143, 144, 145, 147, 148, 149, 179, 180, 193, 197
feelings, 42, 69, 110, 123, 133, 147, 160, 162, 178
finance, 89
financial, x, 2, 89, 95, 96, 99
financial support, 96, 99
food, xviii, 7, 12, 15, 17, 18, 19, 21, 22, 23, 24, 25, 26, 28, 30, 31, 32, 33, 34, 87, 97, 98, 130, 135, 138, 149, 151, 153, 154, 156, 157, 158, 159, 160, 161, 162, 164, 166, 167, 168, 169, 170, 171, 179, 180
food industry, 158
food production, 12, 17, 166
food products, 87, 98, 138
food programs, 18, 31, 149, 170
formal education, 140
foundations, x, 3, 5, 8, 191
fragments, xvii, 66, 108, 109
France, 62, 107, 171, 201
friend, xv, 6, 39, 41, 42, 43, 48, 49, 50, 51, 52, 53, 54, 56, 57, 69
friendship, 49, 51, 54, 69, 74
funds, ix, 20, 24, 25, 28

G

garbage, 129, 130, 183
genetic predisposition, 91
geometry, 69, 174, 186, 194
governments, ix, 2, 4, 18, 19

Greater Buenos Aires, 126, 134, 135, 144, 189
growth, 85, 86, 87, 89, 90
growth rate, 89
Guattari, 116, 122
Guattari, Félix, 115
guidelines, 4, 27, 157, 176
guilt, 24, 167
guilty, 43, 44, 159, 162, 166

H

habitat, 120, 130
health, ix, x, xiv, xv, 3, 9, 10, 18, 21, 22, 30, 31, 34, 39, 40, 41, 44, 50, 59, 60, 91, 95, 98, 127, 128, 130, 134, 135, 136, 168, 169, 170, 174, 176, 182, 183, 184, 186, 187, 188, 189, 190, 191, 193, 196
health care, 182, 184, 187
health services, 130
Heidegger, 120, 122
higher education, 89, 140, 141
history, 3, 22, 24, 64, 142, 171, 175
homes, 127, 128, 129, 159, 180, 183
household income, 130
housing, 97, 127, 130, 136, 144
human, xiv, 2, 3, 5, 6, 13, 14, 15, 39, 46, 48, 80, 81, 91, 109, 111, 112, 113, 114, 116, 117, 118, 120, 121, 122, 128, 135, 157, 169, 174, 175, 176, 185, 188, 194
human actions, 117
human body, 112, 118
human brain, 48
human dignity, 188
human health, 128
human nature, 80, 114
human remains, 188
hunger, v, xiv, xviii, 6, 11, 12, 13, 14, 15, 16, 17, 18, 19, 24, 25, 29, 30, 32, 34, 36, 37, 151, 180
hygiene, 25, 97, 135, 183
hypothesis, 43, 116, 176

I

identification, 42, 69
identity, 14, 52, 102, 148, 181
imaginary, xiii, 25, 78, 107, 108, 111, 113, 118, 201
immune system, 44, 51
immunity, xv, 40, 44, 45, 46, 47, 48, 51, 53
immunization, xv, 6, 39, 40, 41, 42, 44, 46, 47, 48, 49, 50, 51, 52, 53, 54
immunological memory, 44
income, 85, 86, 97, 129, 131, 137, 138, 147, 158
income transfers, 137
individual action, 24, 68
individual hunger, 14
individualism, vii, 158, 166
individuals, 14, 45, 46, 47, 66, 101, 113, 116, 120, 121, 136, 144, 156, 178
industrialization, 144
industries, 85, 90, 98, 99, 100
inequality, 9, 18, 25, 26, 131, 182
infection, 45, 51, 84, 87, 95, 96, 97, 101, 187
infrastructure, 2, 4, 144, 156
institutions, ix, 4, 26, 69, 96, 136, 174
integration, 45, 46, 51, 53, 54, 118, 119
interdependence, 116, 142, 143
intervention, xiv, 12, 13, 26, 29, 30, 68, 135, 136, 137
isolation, xvi, xvii, xviii, 12, 20, 21, 23, 50, 84, 85, 87, 91, 93, 94, 95, 96, 101, 125, 135, 138, 140, 144, 152, 153, 166, 167, 168, 179, 180, 186, 188, 189, 194
issues, 99, 100, 167

K

knowledge, xvii, xviii, 58, 64, 65, 68, 69, 71, 73, 75, 78, 84, 89, 116, 152, 157, 166, 168, 169, 183

L

labor market, 85, 90, 200
labor shortage, 91
labour market, 158
Latin America, vii, 16, 26, 33, 34, 37, 147, 171, 190, 197, 198, 201, 202, 204
learning, xvii, 84, 88, 89, 90, 156, 167
learning activity, 167
learning process, 88
level of education, 139, 141
liberalism, vii, x, 117, 119
life, vii, xiv, 3, 5, 8, 14, 15, 16, 18, 25, 35, 39, 41, 47, 48, 55, 56, 66, 80, 81, 94, 95, 98, 107, 108, 109, 110, 111, 112, 113, 114, 115, 116, 117, 118, 119, 120, 121, 122, 123, 129, 132, 133, 135, 136, 137, 138, 142, 143, 144, 147, 152, 154, 156, 158, 160, 162, 167, 168, 175, 179, 184, 198
light, 42, 165, 186
lived experience, 114, 117, 121
living conditions, 95, 127, 130, 131, 139, 140
loans, 97, 98, 100
logic of Imitation, 71, 74
logistics, 21, 25, 85, 99
loneliness, 91, 194
love, viii, 27, 69, 74, 133, 194, 196

M

Maffesoli, 110, 115, 116, 123
magnitude, 16, 21, 22, 174, 193
management, xvii, 10, 12, 25, 37, 64, 65, 77, 84, 87, 89, 101, 104, 145, 156, 168, 169, 174, 175, 179, 183, 187, 192, 194
market access, viii
market failure, 132
market segment, 89, 158
market stagnation, 6
media, xvi, 20, 28, 41, 60, 61, 62, 63, 64, 66, 92, 93, 104, 108, 117, 174
medical, 84, 88, 100, 101, 102, 129, 130, 174, 182, 184, 188, 191
message, 67, 185, 189
messages, xv, 6, 59, 61, 63, 68, 71, 74, 75, 92, 185
metamorphosis, 27, 78, 145
militarization, 13, 19, 29, 31, 112
military, 21, 26, 41, 180
modernity, 143, 158, 166, 170
modernization, 87, 158
mortality, 180, 182, 193, 194

N

national borders, 4
National Food Program, 17, 32
national security, 23
nature, 9, 55, 74, 80, 109, 112, 114, 115, 117, 118, 119, 120, 157, 169, 187, 193
neoliberalism, vii, x, 5, 117, 119
netizen, 110
nutrients, 13, 14, 15, 19, 154, 155, 156, 168, 169
nutrition, 15, 18, 167
nutritional sensibilities, 168

O

obsessive-compulsive disorder, 91
online survey, xvii, xviii, 7, 86, 126, 134, 152, 153
opportunities, 31, 66, 115, 132

organ, viii, 66, 168
organism, 40, 41, 44, 46, 51, 155
organize, xviii, 16, 29, 77, 110, 152, 156, 164, 168

P

pain, viii, 36, 137, 171, 176, 181, 186
palliative, 186, 191, 193
pandemic, v, vi, vii, ix, xiii, xiv, xv, xvii, xviii, xix, 1, 2, 3, 4, 5, 6, 7, 8, 10, 12, 13, 16, 19, 20, 21, 23, 24, 25, 26, 27, 28, 29, 31, 39, 40, 41, 43, 44, 53, 55, 59, 60, 61, 62, 63, 77, 83, 84, 85, 86, 87, 89, 90, 91, 93, 95, 100, 102, 103, 104, 105, 108,109, 110, 112, 113, 115, 116, 117, 119, 120, 121, 125, 126, 128, 130, 134, 135, 137, 144, 151, 153, 164, 165, 167, 169, 173, 174, 175, 179, 180, 182, 184, 187, 188, 189, 192, 193, 194, 195, 202
pandemic sensibilities, 26
participants, 29, 88, 153, 162, 164
passenger, 96
phenomenology, 117
physical activity, 91
physical education, 98
physical environment, 115, 117
Plan Argentina contra el Hambre, 18
platform, xvi, 60, 62, 65, 66, 77, 79, 90
political crisis, 2, 93
political parties, vii
politics, vii, xviii, 6, 8, 12, 16, 20, 31, 34, 53, 64, 74, 75, 79, 126, 152, 156, 159, 167, 168, 174, 178, 179, 181, 188, 194
politics of bodies, 156, 159, 178, 194
politics of perversion, 31
politics of sensibilities, xviii, 16, 20, 64, 74, 75, 79, 152, 156, 167, 168, 174, 179
pollution, 93, 110
population, xvii, 16, 17, 18, 19, 21, 28, 29, 44, 85, 92, 95, 100, 125, 126, 128, 129, 131, 134, 135, 136, 137, 138, 139, 140, 141, 144, 162, 179, 182
population density, 127
population size, 92
porosity, 110, 113, 115, 118, 119
post-apocalyptic appearance, 110
post-covid city, 118
poverty, ix, xiv, xvi, xvii, 12, 13, 16, 17, 18, 22, 26, 29, 34, 35, 83, 126, 130, 131, 134, 135, 138, 139, 140, 142, 144, 197, 201
prevention, xviii, 101, 135, 151, 176, 188, 192
project, xiv, 1, 24, 89, 118, 119, 128, 184
proposition, 114, 115, 116, 118, 119, 120
protection, viii, 4, 28, 40, 44, 47
proximity, xvii, 52, 80, 108, 109, 114, 119, 174, 178

Q

quarantine, 22, 29, 44, 84, 86, 87, 89, 95, 96, 127, 131, 134, 135, 137, 138, 139, 141, 142, 144, 164, 165, 174, 180
questionnaire, 129, 134

R

reactions, 101, 117
reality, 14, 27, 29, 56, 57, 111, 112, 113, 116, 117, 118, 119, 120, 121, 135, 152, 169
reasoning, vii, xv, 6, 39
recommendations, iv, 187, 188, 189, 191
relatives, 90, 185, 188, 189, 190, 191
reproduction, 13, 14, 16, 19, 30, 64, 68, 74, 132, 133, 154, 156, 157, 168, 169, 179, 181
resource allocation, 12
resources, 15, 16, 21, 29, 132

response, xvi, 3, 18, 44, 50, 51, 83, 88, 118, 134, 142, 143, 144, 178
responsibility, iv, 29, 68, 71, 78
restrictions, xiv, xvi, 1, 84, 95, 114, 134, 192
road transport, 98
Russia, 62, 84, 85, 86, 87, 88, 90, 92, 93, 94, 95, 96, 97, 99, 102, 104, 199
Russian Federation, v, xvi, 7, 83, 84, 95, 96, 97
Russian government, xvi, 83, 84, 98, 100, 104, 105

S

s+c+c, 30
S+I+E, 30
sadness, 108, 137, 148, 186
safety, 49, 101, 102, 107
Saint Petersburg, 84
schedules, 164
school, ix, 29, 88, 114, 139, 158, 167, 180, 199
schooling, 130
science, 3, 29, 45, 108, 111, 201
self-reflection, 15
self-sufficient, 118
seminars, 200
sensation, 64, 69, 116, 144, 155
sensations, 36, 64, 69, 71, 74, 75, 76, 78, 79, 80, 113, 115, 136, 149, 155, 156, 171, 177, 178, 192, 194
senses, 34, 77, 78, 113, 177
sensibilites, 153
sensible, xvii, 108, 109, 115, 117, 118, 119, 120, 121
services, iv, 84, 88, 90, 97, 98, 127, 144, 184, 185
smart city, 118
social assistance, xvii, 35, 126
social construct, 112, 144, 154, 177
social energy, 15, 178
social environment, 48, 116, 194
social fabric, 132
social food policies, 17
social group, 47, 132
social hunger, 14
social institutions, 96
social interaction, 6, 174
social life, vii, 108, 112, 113, 115, 119
social movements, 127
social network, xv, 12, 26, 28, 59, 61, 63, 65, 66, 67, 71, 75, 76, 77, 86, 93, 127, 174, 185, 192
social policies, vi, xviii, 34, 125, 126, 131, 132, 133, 136, 145, 146, 147, 149, 197, 201
social programs, 127, 130, 131, 134, 136, 138, 144, 145
social reality, 112, 113, 116, 117, 119
social regulation, 133, 143
social relations, 66, 112, 115, 142, 154, 157, 168
social relationships, 154, 168
social situations, 133
social structure, 13, 159, 182
social support, xvi, 83, 97, 136, 142
social, preventive and mandatory isolation, xvii, 125
socialization, 117, 156, 158, 176
society, v, vii, viii, x, xiii, xiv, 1, 2, 3, 5, 6, 10, 12, 14, 18, 26, 28, 32, 35, 36, 37, 47, 48, 64, 66, 69, 78, 81, 93, 105, 117, 120, 129, 132, 133, 142, 145, 149, 154, 155, 156, 169, 171, 172, 178, 181, 184, 186, 198, 199, 201, 204
sociocultural contexts, 136
sociology, xix, 3, 5, 6, 9, 12, 14, 64, 65, 78, 110, 111, 145, 148, 154, 173, 176, 177, 193, 201
sociology of bodies, xix, 6, 12, 14, 148, 149, 154, 171, 173, 193
solidarity, 5, 20, 27, 28, 69, 71, 73, 74, 120

Spain, xviii, 62, 152, 153, 162, 163, 164, 165, 166, 183, 197, 203, 204
Spanish flu, xix, 8, 135, 173, 175, 179, 181, 183, 194, 195
spatial segmentation, 127
spatiality, 117
specific knowledge, xviii, 152
spectacle, x, xiii, 5, 8, 26, 27
state of alarm and confinement, 152
state of emergency, xiii
states, x, xiv, 1, 4, 7, 15, 25, 52, 64, 136, 155, 156, 178, 180, 190
street, 29, 109, 110, 112, 115, 121, 129, 131
stress, 64, 91, 149, 165
structure, xvii, 12, 22, 45, 46, 47, 64, 75, 108, 109, 112, 113, 115, 132, 133, 142, 152, 158, 177, 181, 194
structuring, 14, 15, 18, 93, 132, 134, 135, 136, 142, 155, 156, 158, 169, 176, 182, 193, 194, 195
subjective hunger, 14
surveillance, 4, 112, 117

T

target population, 19, 145
target populations, 145
tax collection, 127
taxes, viii, 99
territory, xvii, 80, 116, 126, 129, 183, 186
terrorism, x, xiii, 6, 41, 43
Thomas,William Isaac, 115
time/space management, 168, 179
tourism, 9, 10, 85, 98, 203
training, xvii, 84, 87, 101, 152, 200
transformations, 16, 94, 113, 169, 176, 184
transport, xiii, 3, 85, 98, 180, 182, 183
treatment, 101, 129, 148, 176, 187, 188, 192, 193, 194

U

unemployment rate, 86
universities, ix, 23, 88, 201
urban, x, xvii, 2, 7, 17, 108, 109, 110, 111, 112, 113, 114, 115, 116, 117, 118, 119, 120, 121, 122, 126, 201
urban areas, 2
urban life, 110, 111, 114, 120
urbanity, 108, 113, 115, 116, 117, 118, 119, 121
urbanology, 116

V

valorization, 67, 118, 121, 156
victims, viii, xiii, xiv, 39, 192
violence, vii, ix, xiv, 1, 66, 77, 142, 144
vision, xvii, 14, 78, 108, 109, 117, 121, 132
volunteer, 100, 101, 102
vulnerability, x, xvii, 3, 120, 125, 127, 131, 137

W

war, xi, xiv, 6, 20, 28, 39, 40, 41, 43, 53, 54, 56, 195
water, 21, 127, 128, 144
web, 63, 108, 110, 111, 189
welfare, xvi, 18, 83, 132, 148
well-being, 95, 117, 120, 137, 159, 162, 167
work activity, 129, 137, 144
work environment, 65
workers, 23, 65, 66, 90, 96, 102, 131, 170
workforce, 4

working conditions, 84, 127
working population, 129
worldwide, vii, xiv, 3, 5, 14, 17, 34, 39, 44

Y

young people, xviii, 152, 153, 159, 161, 162, 163, 167, 169